Practical Lipid Management

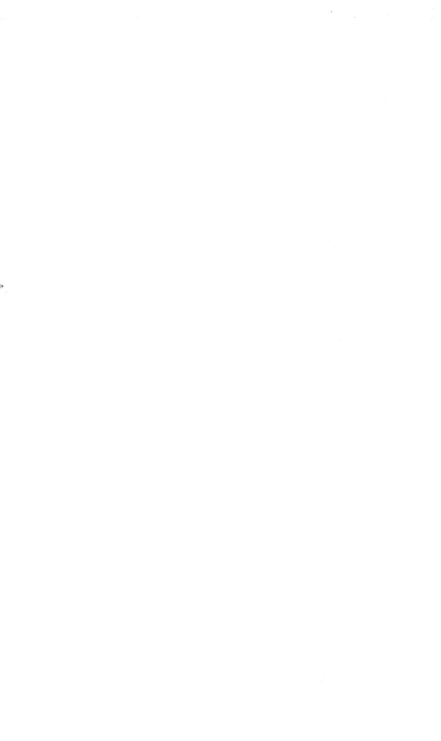

Practical Lipid Management:
Concepts and Controversies

PETER P. TOTH, M.D., PH.D.
Director of Preventive Cardiology
Sterling Rock Falls Clinic, Ltd.
Chief of Medicine, CGH Medical Center
Sterling, Illinois
Clinical Associate Professor
Departments of Family and Community Medicine
University of Illinois College of Medicine
Peoria, Illinois
Southern Illinois University School of Medicine
Springfield, Illinois

KEVIN C. MAKI, PH.D.
President & Chief Science Officer
Provident Clinical Research & Consulting, Inc.
Glen Ellyn, Illinois and Bloomington, Indiana

WILEY-BLACKWELL
A John Wiley & Sons, Ltd., Publication

Library of Congress Cataloging-in-Publication Data

Toth, Peter P.
 Practical lipid management : concepts and controversies / Peter P. Toth,
Kevin C. Maki.
   p. ; cm.
 Includes bibliographical references and index.
 ISBN 978-0-470-05690-5
 1. Hyperlipidemia – Treatment. 2. Coronary heart disease – Prevention. I.
Maki, Kevin C. II. Title.
 [DNLM: 1. Dyslipidemias – therapy. 2. Cardiovascular
Diseases – prevention & control. WD 200.5.H8 T717p 2008]
  RC632.H87T68 2008
  616.3'997 – dc22
                                              2008024773

ISBN: 978-0-470-05690-5

A catalogue record for this book is available from the British Library

Typeset in 9/10.5 Times by Laserwords Private Limited, Chennai, India
Printed in Great Britain by T.J. International Ltd., Padstow, Cornwall.

Contents

Foreword

The critical role of lipid management in the prevention of atherosclerotic disease and its various clinical sequelae is one of the most intensively studied issues in modern medicine. Cholesterol and lipid metabolism are complex and impact the structure and function of cellular organelles, tissue types and whole biological organisms. The circuitry of lipoprotein metabolism and the intricate roles of the gastrointestinal tract and the liver in cholesterol and lipid handling are reasonably well understood. Atherogenesis involves complex interactions among lipoproteins, inflammatory and oxidative mediators, and a variety of cell types, which conspire to induce the formation of foam cells, fatty streaks, and atheromatous plaques in the vasculature. By therapeutically modulating lipoprotein metabolism with drugs such as statins, fibrates, nicotinic acid and fish oils, the development and rate of progression of atherosclerotic disease can be delayed.

A variety of guidelines have been promulgated for lipid management throughout the world. These guidelines are evidence based and incorporate data from epidemiologic investigation, clinical trials, and a variety of other studies (both basic scientific and observational) to derive best practice recommendations. Guidelines are quite consistent in emphasizing the need to reduce serum concentrations of atherogenic lipoproteins such as low-density and very low-density lipoproteins and increase circulating levels of high-density lipoproteins, a class of lipoprotein believed to be anti-atherogenic. Combinations of lifestyle modification and pharmacologic intervention are frequently required to help patients at risk attain their various lipoprotein goals. Compliance with guidelines routinely falls short of stated targets, especially among patients at high risk for acute cardiovascular events. This is despite the fact that aggressive lipid management is consistently associated with significant reductions in risk for cardiovascular events, including myocardial infarction, stroke, and death.

Practical Lipid Management: Concepts and Controversies fills an important gap in the literature. Drs Toth and Maki have written a concise, lucid textbook that is true to its title: a book that is practical, yet also addresses key concepts and controversies in the relationships between various lipids and risk for cardiovascular disease. This book is designed for the busy clinician who needs authoritative information in a user-friendly format. In addition to covering key management issues associated with specific forms of dyslipidemia, the authors carefully detail the mechanistic basis of atherogenesis, the epidemiologic investigations that elucidated

the relationship between lipids and atherosclerotic disease, the evolution of
the National Cholesterol Education Program's Adult Treatment Panel, risk
assessment, the design and interpretation of clinical trials, the role of lipid
management in women and racial minorities, and the use of emerging risk
factors and biomarkers. Illustrative case studies emphasizing the variety of
dyslipidemias one can expect to encounter in primary care and suggested
approaches to their management are also provided. A feature of this textbook
is the presentation of a series of "sidebars", which critically and insightfully
appraise several controversies in modern lipid management.

The stated goal of this book is to improve patient care among patients
afflicted with dyslipidemia. The health care providers who read and apply
the contents of this excellent, practical textbook will certainly be empowered
to achieve this objective.

Christopher P. Cannon, M.D.

TIMI Study Group
Brigham and Women's Hospital
Harvard Medical School
Boston, MA
USA

Preface

The US National Cholesterol Education Program (NCEP) Adult Treatment Panel I Guidelines for the Detection, Evaluation and Treatment of High Cholesterol were published in 1988 and have since undergone two major and several less comprehensive updates. Since the time that the first large, randomized clinical event trials were published showing that cholesterol lowering with medication reduced cardiovascular events, an enormous body of literature has evolved that has continued to support the critical role of dyslipidemia management in the prevention of atherosclerotic disease and its consequences, including myocardial infarction and acute coronary syndromes, stroke, intermittent claudication, and mortality.

Lipid and sterol metabolism involve highly evolved biochemical pathways and regulatory circuitry of great complexity. Lipids are crucial to the structural and functional integrity of all mammalian cell types. Numerous lipid species are involved in cell signaling, formation of specialized membrane domains, and serve as oxidizable substrate in intermediary metabolism, among many other functions. Lipoproteins have evolved as highly specialized transport vehicles of lipids and sterols in aqueous media. When present in excess, the lipids and sterols in lipoproteins are pathogenic and constitute key potentiators of atherosclerotic disease.

As insights into the pathophysiologies of various dyslipidemias and their relationships to atherothrombosis have become further refined, so too has the complexity of the guidelines for lipid management. The current recommendations recognize five risk categories and include primary, secondary, tertiary, and optional treatment goals. These guidelines continue to emphasize the enormous need for aggressive, sustained lifestyle modification in patients with dyslipidemia; they introduced the concept of non-high-density lipoprotein cholesterol (non-HDL-C); a new definition for the metabolic syndrome; defined five clinical entities as coronary heart disease (CHD) risk equivalents; emphasized the need for Framingham risk scoring for stratifying patient risk; and redefined the threshold for what constitutes a low serum HDL-C. Fortunately, the number of drugs in our therapeutic armamentarium has expanded with the addition of new classes of medications for altering the lipid profile allowing the clinician to help more people than ever before to maintain lipid levels within the recommended ranges. Several promising classes of lipid modifying drugs are currently in late-stage development. Many of these will allow clinicians to more specifically target therapies towards specific molecular lesions and metabolic impairments of lipoprotein metabolism.

Although it is difficult to overstate the importance of sound lipid management, clinicians are faced with a daunting collection of options and recommendations to keep track of and apply, not only for evaluation and treatment of lipid disorders, but also for other conditions including hypertension, diabetes, asthma, various cancers, and a variety of other commonly encountered medical issues. In the authors' experience, interest in lipid management and the desire to follow current treatment recommendations are high, but busy clinicians are overwhelmed by the amount of information that must be committed to memory. Further complicating this is the fact that the number of cardiovascular clinical trials in progress at any given time is staggering. Keeping up with the flow of this much information is extremely challenging to absorb and to apply in daily clinical practice.

When speaking to clinicians about lipid management, particularly those in primary care, the authors have repeatedly been asked to recommend a book that includes a concise, user-friendly overview of the lipid management process, while providing balanced and informed perspectives on issues about which expert opinion is divided or rapidly evolving. *Practical Lipid Management: Concepts and Controversies* is an attempt to provide such a source of information to a target audience that includes primary care clinicians (physicians, advanced practice nurses, physician assistants), as well as clinicians in training, pharmacists, and dietitians.

The need for increased clinician education about dyslipidemia management was demonstrated by a national survey of lipid management in clinical practice in 2003. This survey, the National Cholesterol Education Program Evaluation Project Utilizing Novel E-technology II (NEPTUNE II), confirmed that several treatment gaps exist between current recommendations and results obtained in clinical practice, particularly with regard to the features of the NCEP guidelines that are relatively new. For example, the concept of CHD risk equivalents and the inclusion of non-HDL-C treatment targets were added to the NCEP guidelines in 2001. Among patients categorized as having CHD risk equivalents in NEPTUNE II, low-density lipoprotein cholesterol (LDL-C) goal achievement ranged from 55% among patients with diabetes to only 40% among those with other CHD risk equivalents. Furthermore, in patients with triglycerides ≥ 200 mg dl^{-1} (one-quarter of the study sample), only 17–33% of those in the CHD and risk equivalents subcategories had achieved both their LDL-C and non-HDL-C goals.

While the results from NEPTUNE II show substantial improvement compared with those from a similar previous survey (the Lipid Treatment Assessment Programme) that was completed in 1997, a great deal of room for improvement still exists. This is especially true in light of updated treatment recommendations that emphasize the value of even more aggressive optional targets for LDL-C and non-HDL-C for patients in newly created "very high risk" and "moderately high risk" categories. The authors believe that *Practical Lipid Management* will be a useful tool for clinicians seeking to enhance their skills and knowledge in this area. The diagnosis and management of dyslipidemias constitutes the cornerstone for preventing cardiovascular events in both the primary and secondary settings. It is our sincere wish that this book will heighten awareness of the importance of lipid management and contribute meaningfully to the prevention of atherosclerotic disease and its many clinical sequelae.

Peter P. Toth, MD, PhD
Sterling Rock Falls Clinic
Sterling, Illinois, USA

Kevin C. Maki, PhD
Provident Clinical Research
Glen Ellyn, Illinois, USA

Acknowledgements

We would like to express gratitude to the following staff of Provident Clinical Research & Consulting, Inc. for their hard work and diligence in the preparation of this manuscript: Serena Hess, Theresa Tardi, Dr Tia Rains and Barbara Anderson. We thank Jude Gonzalez for rendering the color figures and Jennifer Taber for administrative assistance. The authors also thank Dr Joan Marsh and Fiona Woods (John Wiley & Sons) for their support of this book.

1 Epidemiology of Lipids, Lipid Management and Risk for Coronary Heart Disease: An Overview

Key Points

- *Epidemiological studies have shown that a large percentage of the variation within and between countries in coronary heart disease (CHD) incidence can be accounted for by lipid-associated risk factors.*

- *More than 90% of the population-attributable risk for CHD can be explained by potentially modifiable risk factors (lipids, blood pressure, body weight, diabetes, psychosocial factors, diet, and physical activity).*

- *Clinical trials have shown that each 1% reduction in low-density lipoprotein cholesterol (LDL-C) is associated with a reduction of approximately 1% in CHD risk. However, observational data suggest that the benefit may be as much as 3% CHD risk reduction per 1% decrement in LDL-C if maintained for many years.*

- *The non-high-density lipoprotein cholesterol (non-HDL-C) level is highly correlated with the level of apolipoprotein B and is a better predictor of CHD risk than LDL-C in patients with elevated triglycerides (≥ 200 mg dl^{-1}); therefore non-HDL-C goals have been established by the National Cholesterol Education Program (NCEP) as secondary targets for patients with elevated triglycerides.*

- *National surveys indicate that cholesterol management in clinical practice has improved dramatically since 1997, although recent research shows some groups are at increased risk for not achieving their*

Practical Lipid Management: Concepts and Controversies   Peter P. Toth and Kevin C. Maki
© 2008 John Wiley & Sons, Ltd

treatment targets, including patients with elevated triglycerides, women, minorities, current smokers, and those with CHD risk equivalents.

- *Based on recently published evidence that reducing LDL-C to levels well below 100 mg dl^{-1} is associated with further reductions in risk, the NCEP has issued optional treatment targets for patients at very high risk, including LDL-C < 70 mg dl^{-1}.*

- *It is likely that use of high-dose statin and multidrug therapy will need to expand in order to achieve these more aggressive goals.*

1.1 EARLY HISTORY OF CARDIOVASCULAR EPIDEMIOLOGY

As recently as 1950, the prevailing view in the medical community was that atherosclerosis was a degenerative condition that was an inevitable result of aging. In the early 1950s, Ancel Keys and colleagues documented that mortality from CHD varied enormously between countries [1]. The results of the Seven Countries Study showed that coronary mortality differed by roughly 10-fold between countries and that the average circulating cholesterol level was strongly associated with coronary death [1, 2]. Later studies showed that when groups of people migrated from developing countries to more developed western countries, and adopted lifestyle features of their new home, their blood cholesterol levels rose and this was accompanied by an increase in CHD [3]. These findings were supported by results from early autopsy studies that showed marked variation in cholesterol levels and coronary atherosclerosis between countries [1].

The Framingham Heart Study was initiated in 1948 and provided the foundation for the idea that variation in CHD rates within a population could be predicted by several "risk factors". In fact, the term *risk factor* was first used in 1961 in a publication from this landmark investigation, which measured various characteristics of a group of roughly 5000 residents in the town of Framingham, Massachusetts and followed them over decades to determine what features were associated with CHD and other cardiovascular events.

Epidemiology is the study of the distribution and determinants of disease in human populations. Before the middle of the twentieth century, epidemiological methods had mainly been employed in the study of infectious diseases ("epidemics"). The Framingham Heart Study has contributed hundreds of papers to the scientific literature that helped to establish the risk factors that were associated with the development of CHD. Many of these were identifiable years or decades before clinical events, suggesting the potential for prevention through risk factor modification.

Thus, the foundation laid by the study of risk factors associated with variations in CHD incidence between and within populations has allowed the development of clinical tools for risk stratification, such as the Framingham Risk Score, that has been incorporated into the NCEP guidelines [4]. A central feature of the approach advocated by the NCEP is matching the intensity of lipid modification with the level of CHD risk. The NCEP method entails use of major CHD risk factors (sex, age, HDL-C, smoking status, blood pressure, diabetes) and the presence or absence of clinical atherosclerosis to stratify subjects according to 10-year CHD risk. Specific treatment goals for LDL-C are recommended, with those at the highest risk (known CHD or risk equivalents) having the most aggressive goals.

1.2 LIPID RISK FACTORS ARE CENTRAL TO EFFORTS AT CHD PREVENTION

Recently, the INTERHEART study evaluated the relationships between major risk factors identified in earlier epidemiologic investigations and CHD in 52 countries [5]. This global investigation showed that nine potentially modifiable risk factors could explain more than 90% of the variation in acute myocardial infarction among men and women (Table 1.1).

The results from INTERHEART illustrate the importance of lipid-related risk factors. Because of its strong association with CHD risk and high prevalence, an elevated ratio of apolipoprotein B to AI explains nearly half (49.2%) of the global population-attributable risk for CHD. Apolipoprotein B is the main protein constituent of atherogenic lipoproteins (LDL, very low-density lipoprotein (VLDL), and remnants of triglyceride-rich particles), whereas apolipoprotein AI is the main protein constituent of HDL, which is inversely associated with CHD risk. Accordingly, these apolipoprotein concentrations indicate the number of circulating atherogenic (apolipoprotein B) and protective (apolipoprotein AI) lipoprotein particles.

Clinically, lipoprotein cholesterol levels are more commonly measured than apolipoproteins. Many studies have shown that levels of non-HDL-C and HDL-C are highly correlated with apolipoprotein B and AI levels, respectively, and have predictive values that are only slightly less robust than those of apolipoproteins [6]. The NCEP ATP III guidelines have recommended the use of lipoprotein cholesterol (LDL, non-HDL and HDL) and triglyceride concentrations for assessment of CHD risk status. Treatment goals have been recommended for LDL-C as the primary target of lipid management, and non-HDL-C as a secondary target for patients with elevated triglycerides (≥ 200 mg dl^{-1}). Treatment targets are discussed in detail in Chapter 3.

Table 1.1 Potentially modifiable risk factors, their association with coronary heart disease case status and estimated population-attributable risk in the INTERHEART study.

Category	Variable	Odds ratio[a]	Population-attributable risk (%)[b]
1. Lipids	Apo[c] B/Apo AI ratio	3.25	49.2
2. Smoking	Current, past, never	2.87	35.7
3. Psychosocial factors	Composite	2.67	32.5
4. Abdominal obesity	Waist hip ratio	1.62	20.1
5. History of hypertension	Yes, no	1.91	17.9
6. Fruit and vegetable intake	Frequency	0.70	13.7
7. Physical activity	Frequency	0.86	12.2
8. Diabetes mellitus	Yes, no	2.37	9.9
9. Alcohol intake	Frequency	0.91	6.7
Total			90.4

[a]Estimated from a logistic regression model adjusted for age, sex and all other variables. Comparisons for odds ratios were as follows: apolipoprotein B/AI ratio, top versus lowest quintile; smoking, current versus never; psychosocial factors, index for depression, general stress, low locus of control, major life events, versus nonexposure to all five factors; abdominal obesity, top versus bottom tertile; hypertension and diabetes history, yes versus no; physical activity, ≥4 hours per week versus <4 hours per week; alcohol consumption ≥3 times per week versus <3 times per week; daily fruit and vegetable intake versus none or irregular.
[b]Population-attributable risk is the percentage of cases that can be attributed to this risk factor given the probability of exposure in the population and the increase or decrease in relative risk (or relative odds) associated with the risk factor.
[c]Apo, apolipoprotein.
Adapted from Yusuf *et al.* (2004) *Lancet*, **364**, 937–52, [5] with permission from Elsevier.

1.3 LDL-C AND CHD RISK

LDL particles typically carry a majority of the circulating cholesterol and evidence from population, laboratory and intervention studies has clearly shown that these particles are atherogenic. Populations that maintain LDL-C <100 mg dl^{-1} have very low rates of CHD. The average LDL-C concentration among adults in the United States of America (USA) is ~123 mg dl^{-1} [7]. Therefore, a majority of the population can be considered to have some increase in CHD risk due to elevation in LDL-C, which accounts, in part, for the high lifetime risk for clinical CHD in the USA: 49% for men and 32% for women [8]. When other consequences of atherosclerotic disease (e.g. stroke, peripheral arterial disease, and revascularization procedures) are considered, it becomes evident that a majority of Americans can be expected to suffer from clinical atherosclerotic disease at some time in their lives. Lifetime risk for cardiovascular disease is approximately two in three for men and one in two for women in the USA [9].

A strong linear relationship exists between the level of LDL-C and CHD risk that is independent of other major CHD risk factors. Clinical trials of interventions for lowering LDL-C have consistently shown reduced CHD events after various treatments to lower LDL-C including diet, ileal bypass surgery, and drug therapy with bile acid sequestrant and statin drugs [4]. Meta-analyses [4, 10, 11] indicate that benefits are observed in all subgroups studied, including those with or without prior evidence of atherosclerotic disease, in the presence or absence of other risk factors such as diabetes or hypertension, and at all baseline levels of lipids and lipoproteins. Recent studies suggest that the relationship between LDL-C and CHD event rate extends to LDL-C levels well below 100 mg dl^{-1} (Figure 1.1), which prompted the NCEP to recommend an optional LDL-C treatment goal of <70 mg dl^{-1} for patients at "very high risk" [12, 13].

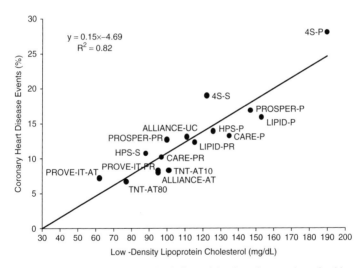

Figure 1.1 Low-density lipoprotein cholesterol levels and proportion of subjects with coronary heart disease events in secondary prevention trials. 4S, scandinavian simvastatin survival study; ALLIANCE, aggressive lipid-lowering initiation abates new cardiac events trial; AT, atorvastatin (10 or 80 mg); CARE, cholesterol and recurrent events trial; HPS, heart protection study; LIPID, long-term intervention with pravastatin in ischemic disease trial; P, placebo; PR, pravastatin; PROSPER, prospective study of pravastatin in the elderly at risk; PROVE-IT, pravastatin or atorvastatin evaluation and infection therapy trial; R^2, coefficient of determination; S, simvastatin; TNT, treating to new targets trial; UC, usual care. From Maki, K.C. *et al.* (2005) *The American Journal of Cardiology*, **96** (suppl 9A), 59K–64K, [13] with permission from Elsevier.

1.4   LDL-C LOWERING AND CHD RISK REDUCTION

Clinical trial results have shown that each 1% reduction in LDL-C reduces CHD event risk by roughly 1% over a period of five years. However, atherosclerotic disease develops and progresses over decades. Accordingly, trials of three to six years may be insufficient to demonstrate the full benefit of LDL-C lowering. Evidence from observational studies suggests that the benefits may be larger if reduced LDL-C concentrations are maintained over an extended period. For example, Cohen *et al.* [14] studied the effects of mutations in a protease gene involved in LDL receptor degradation on LDL-C levels and CHD events in the Atherosclerosis Risk in Communities study. They found that a version of the mutation that was associated with a 28% lower LDL-C level was also associated with a remarkable 88% reduction in the incidence of CHD. Another mutation that was associated with a 15% lower level of LDL-C was associated with a 47% reduction in the incidence of CHD. These findings, as well as inter-country comparisons,

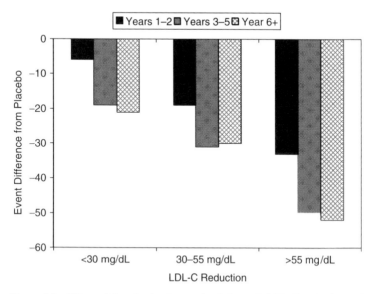

Figure 1.2   Effects of low-density lipoprotein cholesterol (LDL-C) reduction and length of treatment on the difference from placebo in ischemic heart disease events based on a meta-analysis of 50 trials of lipid modification with at least one year of treatment. Adapted from Law, M.R. *et al.* (2003) *British Medical Journal*, **326**, 1423–30 [10] with permission from BMJ Publishing Group.

suggest that each 1% lowering of LDL-C might produce a 2–3% reduction in CHD risk if maintained over an extended period [2]. Clinical trial results provide some support for this concept, in that they have generally shown greater risk reduction with longer treatment (Figure 1.2), although few trials have extended beyond six years, limiting the conclusions that can be drawn from the available data.

In the past a great deal of debate has surrounded the question of how aggressively LDL-C should be managed in elderly patients. One reason for this was that the relative risk increase for an elevated level of LDL cholesterol in epidemiological studies was smaller in the elderly than in younger subjects. However, the benefits of preventive therapies depend not only on the relative risk reduction that can be achieved, but also on the absolute risk of the individual for the event. For example, if the relative risk reduction associated with a 30% lowering of LDL-C in a younger individual is 30%, but only two-thirds of that (20%) in an elderly individual, the absolute risk reduction is larger for the older patient because of the higher baseline risk. Average 10-year risk for a 72-year-old man in the USA is ~25%, whereas that for a 45-year-old man is ~6%. A 20% reduction for the older man reduces event risk by 5%, whereas a 30% reduction for the younger man reduces absolute event risk by only 1.8%. Therefore, the NCEP treatment goals for LDL-C apply across the age spectrum in adults.

1.5 OTHER ATHEROGENIC LIPOPROTEINS: ATHEROGENIC REMNANTS

While the data supporting the relationship between increased LDL-C and CHD risk are extremely well established, other atherogenic lipoproteins also appear to contribute to CHD risk. For years it has been recognized that elevated levels of triglycerides were associated with increased CHD incidence. However, because the triglyceride concentration varies substantially from day-to-day and hypertriglyceridemia is associated with a number of other risk factors including depressed levels of HDL-C; small, dense LDL particles; and increased levels of inflammatory and hemostatic markers, determining the independent contribution of elevated triglycerides to CHD risk was difficult. In recent years it has become clear that remnants of triglyceride-rich lipoproteins, including VLDL, intermediate-density lipoprotein (IDL), and chylomicron remnant particles, are atherogenic. Although technology exists to measure remnant particles, or the lipids carried by such particles, these are mainly research tools. In clinical practice, the VLDL-C concentration may be used as an indicator of the circulating level of atherogenic remnants and a target for modification.

In patients with triglyceride levels <200 mg dl^{-1}, a large majority of the cholesterol carried by atherogenic particles is carried by LDL particles. Therefore, the primary therapeutic strategy is to maintain LDL-C at an acceptable level for the patient's CHD risk status. However, when the triglyceride level is elevated (≥ 200 mg dl^{-1}), levels of atherogenic remnants are also increased, thus the LDL-C level alone does not fully account for the burden of circulating atherogenic particles.

Non-HDL-C is calculated as the difference between the total and HDL-C concentrations. It represents all of the cholesterol carried by potentially atherogenic particles containing apolipoprotein B, including LDL, VLDL,

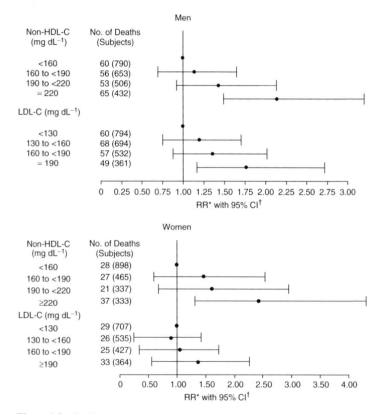

Figure 1.3 Cardiovascular disease mortality by non-high-density lipoprotein cholesterol and low-density lipoprotein cholesterol levels in men and women. RR, relative risk; CI, confidence interval. Adapted from Cui, Y. *et al.* (2001) *Archives of Internal Medicine*, **161**, 1413–19, [15].

IDL, lipoprotein(a), and chylomicron remnant particles. The level of non-HDL-C is highly correlated with the apolipoprotein B concentration, and, like apolipoprotein B, has been found to be a better predictor of cardiovascular mortality than LDL-C (Figure 1.3) [15]. Accordingly, the NCEP ATP III recommended non-HDL-C goals as secondary targets for treatment in patients with elevated triglycerides (≥ 200 mg dl^{-1}). As discussed in Chapter 3, the non-HDL-C goal is 30 mg dl^{-1} above the LDL-C goal for each risk category. Thus, although the triglyceride level is used for classification, treatments goals focus on reductions in lipoprotein cholesterol levels (LDL-C and VLDL-C) rather than on triglycerides *per se*.

1.6 HDL-C AND CHD RISK

Population studies have consistently shown a strong inverse correlation between HDL-C and CHD risk. Each decrement of 1% in HDL-C is associated with an increase of 2–3% in CHD event rate. Evidence from animal studies and from genetic conditions associated with low or high circulating levels of HDL or HDL-C suggests that these particles may play a direct role in atherogenesis. HDL particles are involved in "reverse cholesterol transport," acting to remove cholesterol from peripheral tissues, including foam cells in the arterial wall, and delivering it to the liver for excretion, either directly or via transfer to other lipoproteins (VLDL and LDL).

Although the weight of the evidence suggests that HDL particles are directly antiatherogenic, the mechanisms by which they exert their effects are only partially understood (see Chapter 7 for further discussion). Unlike LDL, no drugs have been tested in outcomes studies that markedly alter the HDL concentration without concomitant effects on other lipoproteins (VLDL and LDL). However, multivariate statistical analyses of results from clinical trials suggest that increases in HDL-C induced by some lipid drugs such as statins and fibrates do contribute to the observed reductions in cardiovascular event rates [4].

Several mechanisms exist through which the HDL-C or HDL particle concentration can be increased, but it is not certain that all will be beneficial. Moreover, the HDL-C concentration is strongly associated with levels of other risk factors such as triglycerides, remnant lipoproteins and small, dense LDL particles. Therefore, the degree to which a reduced HDL or HDL-C level is contributing directly to CHD risk still remains unclear. A low HDL-C concentration (<40 mg dl^{-1}) is counted as a major CHD risk factor for risk stratification, and as a component of the Metabolic Syndrome (<40 mg dl^{-1} for men, <50 mg dl^{-1}L for women) in the NCEP recommendations. Therapeutic efforts to raise HDL-C are via non-drug and drug therapies are advocated for those with low levels, particularly weight loss, increased physical activity, and smoking cessation, where appropriate.

However, the ATP III did not establish HDL-C treatment goals. Risk stratification and identification is covered in detail in Chapter 4.

1.7 TRENDS IN LIPIDS AND LIPID MANAGEMENT IN THE USA

The results of the Lipid Research Clinics Coronary Primary Prevention Trial were published in 1984, which provided the first clear evidence from a randomized clinical trial that lowering the circulating cholesterol level results in a reduction in CHD events [16]. The ATP I recommendations from the NCEP were published in 1988, followed by ATP II in 1993 and ATP III in 2001. A national survey of lipid management in clinical practice called the Lipid Treatment Assessment Program was conducted in 1996 and 1997. Despite the fact that the survey focused on physicians who were high prescribers of lipid-altering drug therapies, the results showed that only 38% of patients overall had achieved their target LDL-C concentration and that only 18% of those with CHD had an LDL-C concentration of 100 mg dl^{-1} or less, as recommended by the ATP II guidelines [17].

Data from the National Health and Nutrition Examination Surveys show that the average serum cholesterol level among men and women 60–74 years of age in the USA declined by more than 9% between the 1976–1980 and 1999–2002 surveys [7]. The fall in average cholesterol level was much larger during this period among older individuals than among younger participants (<40 years), who showed declines of 2–4%. This decline was likely due to a combination of lifestyle changes (e.g. less consumption of saturated fat and cholesterol) and greater use of cholesterol-lowering drug therapies. Between the 1988–1994 and 1999–2002 surveys, the fraction of men 60–74 years of age who reported use of a cholesterol-lowering medication increased from 6.8 to 24.3%. The corresponding numbers for women were 8.7 and 21.6%, respectively. The expanded use of cholesterol-lowering drug therapy corresponded with a period when data from large, randomized clinical trials of lipid-altering interventions, particularly statin drugs, were rapidly accumulating.

1.8 THE NATIONAL CHOLESTEROL EDUCATION PROGRAM EVALUATION PROJECT USING NOVEL E-TECHNOLOGY (NEPTUNE) II SURVEY

In 2003, the NEPTUNE II survey was conducted as a follow-up to the Lipid Treatment Assessment Program. This national survey of patients receiving lipid management from physicians who were high prescribers of lipid-altering drugs showed that 67% of the 4885 subjects had achieved their LDL-C treatment goal, including 62% of those with CHD [18]. These rates of treatment success compared favorably with those from 1997 (38 and 18%, respectively) [17]. However, despite the fact that the survey only included patients of physicians who were high prescribers of lipid-altering medications, and therefore likely to have been managing lipids more effectively than average, several gaps existed between the NCEP ATP III recommendations and what was achieved in practice.

Treatment success was strongly related to risk category (Figure 1.4) [18]. Most subjects (89%) with 0–1 risk factor (LDL-C goal <160 mg dl^{-1}) had achieved their LDL-C goal, whereas only 57% of those with CHD or risk equivalents had achieved their treatment target (LDL-C <100 mg dl^{-1}). Subjects with triglycerides ≥200 mg dl^{-1} were less likely to have achieved their LDL-C target in each risk category. The percentage of subjects who had achieved both their LDL-C and non-HDL-C targets was lower still.

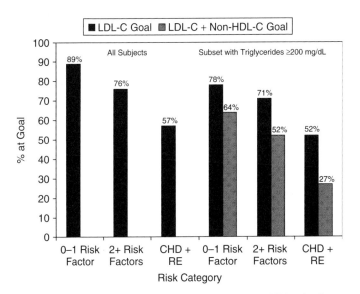

Figure 1.4 Percentage of subjects at their National Cholesterol Education Program Adult Treatment Panel III treatment goals according to risk category for all subjects and the subset with triglycerides >200 mg dl^{-1} in the National Cholesterol Education Program Evaluation Project Utilizing Novel E-technology (NEPTUNE) II survey. LDL-C, low-density lipoprotein cholesterol; non-HDL-C, non-high-density lipoprotein cholesterol; RE, risk equivalent. Adapted from Davidson, M.H. *et al.* (2005) *The American Journal of Cardiology*, **96**, 556–63 [18] with permission of Elsevier.

Notably, only 27% of those with CHD and risk equivalents had achieved their LDL-C and non-HDL-C targets.

Factors associated with a greater likelihood of goal achievement included older age, a greater number of major CHD risk factors, use of drug therapy, use of a high efficacy statin (simvastatin or atorvastatin) and treatment by a subspecialist (cardiology or endocrinology) [18]. In contrast, minority ethnicity, female sex (CHD and risk equivalents category only), current smoking and presence of a non-CHD risk equivalent (diabetes, non-CHD atherosclerosis, or multiple risk factors producing an estimated 10-year CHD risk >20%) were associated with a lower likelihood of goal achievement [18–20]. In addition, fewer than 10% of subjects were taking more than one lipid medication (70% of subjects were on statin monotherapy), which is nearly identical to the prevalence of combination drug use in the Lipid Treatment Assessment Program.

These findings suggest that aspects of the NCEP recommendations that are new to ATP III have not been fully assimilated into clinical practice (e.g. non-HDL-C goals and CHD risk equivalents). They also indicate that women, minorities and smokers are at increased risk for insufficient lipid management and clinicians should target these groups for more aggressive therapy. Furthermore, in light of new evidence showing that the benefits of lipid therapy extend to levels of LDL-C <100 mg dl^{-1}, the NCEP has issued new, more aggressive (but optional) treatment targets [12]. It appears likely that use of high-dose statin and multi-drug therapy will need to expand in order to achieve these more aggressive goals. It is notable that 75% of subjects in the NEPTUNE II study who were in the CHD and risk equivalents category would qualify as "very high risk" and thus be eligible for an optional LDL-C treatment target of <70 mg dl^{-1}.

CONTROVERSY

SHOULD A MEASURE OF ATHEROGENIC LIPOPROTEIN PARTICLE NUMBER BE USED IN RISK ASSESSMENT AND/OR TO EVALUATE THE RESPONSE TO LIPID THERAPY?

In recent years it has become apparent that lipoproteins other than LDL have atherogenic potential. Triglyceride-rich lipoproteins such as VLDL, IDL, and chylomicron remnants have been found to contribute to the development and progression of atherosclerotic plaques in animal models. Furthermore, conditions associated with elevated levels of remnant lipoproteins in the absence of increased LDL-C (e.g. familial dysbetalipoproteinemia) are associated with increased risk for CHD. These findings prompted the NCEP ATP III to establish non-HDL-C as a secondary target for treatment. Non-HDL-C correlates strongly with the circulating concentration of Apo B and represents the cholesterol carried by all types of potentially atherogenic particles, including LDL, lipoprotein(a), and triglyceride-rich lipoproteins.

Since each potentially atherogenic particle contains only one molecule of Apo B, the Apo B concentration provides a measure of the number of circulating particles with atherogenic potential. Some Apo B-containing particles may be more atherogenic than others. For example, LDL particles may be more atherogenic than VLDL particles and smaller, denser LDL particles may be more atherogenic than larger, more buoyant LDL particles. However, the gradient of atherogenicity of Apo B containing particles has not been fully quantified and is the subject of considerable debate (see Chapter 6 for more detail regarding this issue). Nevertheless, several studies have shown that Apo B or non-HDL-C predict CHD events better than LDL-C, particularly when the triglyceride concentration is elevated, lending support to the concept that the number of circulating atherogenic particles is a more precise indicator of dyslipidemia-associated CHD risk than LDL-C [1].

An additional consideration is the influence of drug therapy on lipoprotein cholesterol levels, as compared to the number of circulating atherogenic particles. Figure 1 shows the effects of statin therapy on LDL-C, non-HDL-C, and Apo B concentrations during a large clinical trial, expressed as population percentiles [2]. All three variables had baseline values above the 85th percentile. During statin treatment the mean values for LDL-C and non-HDL-C dropped to roughly the 25th percentile. However, the mean Apo B level was still above the 50th percentile. Thus, statin therapy lowered cholesterol levels relatively more than it lowered the number of atherogenic particles.

A similar conclusion has been reached when the number of LDL particles (LDL-P) was examined with nuclear magnetic resonance in subjects with type 2 diabetes who had LDL-C $<100\,\mathrm{mg\,dl^{-1}}$ (most of whom were likely receiving lipid drug therapy). An LDL-C value of $100\,\mathrm{mg\,dl^{-1}}$ represents approximately the 25th percentile in the US population. Nearly one-quarter (23.7%) of these individuals with LDL-C in the bottom quartile for the population had an LDL-P concentration that was above the 50th percentile ($1300\,\mathrm{nmol\,l^{-1}}$) [3].

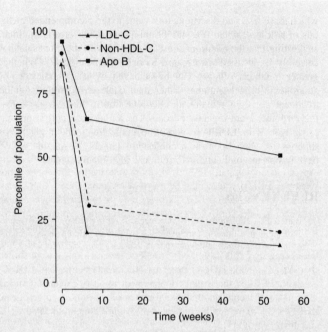

Figure 1 Effects of statin therapy on low density lipoprotein cholesterol (LDL-C), non-high-density lipoprotein cholesterol (non-HDL-C) and
apolipoprotein B (apo B) concentrations, expressed as population percentiles
in the Atorvastatin Comparative Cholesterol Efficacy and Safety Study.
Reprinted from Sniderman, A.D. *et al.* (2003) *Lancet*, **361**, 777–80 [2] with
kind permission of Elsevier.

Taken together, these results suggest that using non-HDL-C and
LDL-C levels to evaluate the effects of treatment can lead to an overestimation of the degree to which atherogenic particle concentration
has been reduced. This raises the possibility that using Apo B or
LDL-P responses would provide the clinician with a better indication
of the degree of risk reduction than relying on lipoprotein cholesterol
levels (LDL-C and non-HDL-C). Of course, using either of these
tests entails added expense and complexity.

The questions of whether use of apolipoproteins or measurements
of particle concentrations add predictive value to risk assessment
has been addressed in several recent studies [4–6]. The results have
uniformly supported greater predictive ability of measures of particle
number compared with lipoprotein levels. However, the degree to

which these tests add discriminatory value to the recommended methods of risk assessment (e.g. the Framingham risk score) is minimal, suggesting that the additional cost associated with these tests cannot currently be justified with regard to risk stratification [7]. Whether greater treatment efficacy can be achieved by using indicators of atherogenic particle number rather than cholesterol levels to guide treatment decisions remains an open question. Clinical trials to test this hypothesis are urgently needed. The authors are optimistic that using Apo B or LDL-P responses to guide treatment might prove superior to using lipoprotein cholesterol targets. If so, this would have important implications for clinical lipid management.

REFERENCES

[1] Barter, P.J., Ballantyne, C.M., Carmena, R. et al. (2006) Apo B versus cholesterol in estimating cardiovascular risk and in guiding therapy: report of the thirty-person/ten-country panel. Journal of Internal Medicine, 259, 247–58.

[2] Sniderman, A.D., Furberg, C.D., Roeters van Lennep, J.E. et al. (2003) Apolipoproteins versus lipids as indices of coronary risk and as targets for statin therapy. Lancet, 361, 777–80.

[3] Cromwell, W.C. and Otvos, J.D. (2006) Heterogeneity of low-density lipoprotein particle number in patients with type 2 diabetes mellitus and low-density lipoprotein cholesterol <100 mg/dl. The American Journal of Cardiology, 98, 1599–602.

[4] Ingelsson, E., Schaefer, E.J., Contois, J.H. et al. (2007) Clinical utility of different lipid measures for prediction of coronary heart disease in men and women. The Journal of the American Medical Association, 298, 776–85.

[5] Van der Steeg, W.A., Boekholdt, S.M., Stein, E.A. et al. (2007) Role of the apolipoprotein-B-apolipoprotein A-I ratio in cardiovascular risk assessment: a case-control analysis in EPIC-Norfolk. Annals of Internal Medicine, 146, 640–48.

[6] Cromwell, W.C., Otvos, J.D., Keyes, M.J. et al. (2007) LDL particle number and risk of future cardiovascular disease in the Framingham Offspring Study – implications for LDL management. Journal of Clinical Lipidology, 1, 583–92.

[7] Berkwits, M. and Guallar, E. (2007) Risk factors, risk prediction, and the apolipoprotein B – apolipoprotein A-I ratio. Annals of Internal Medicine, 146, 677–79.

REFERENCES

[1] Epstein, F.H. (1992) Contribution of epidemiology to understanding coronary heart disease, in Coronary Heart Disease Epidemiology from Aetiology to Public

Health (eds M. Marmot and P. Elliott), Oxford University Press, New York, pp. 20–32.

[2] Brown, B.G., Stukovsky, K.H. and Zhao, X.Q. (2006) Simultaneous low-density lipoprotein-C lowering and high-density lipoprotein-C elevation for optimum cardiovascular disease prevention with various drug classes, and their combinations: a meta-analysis of 23 randomized lipid trials. *Current Opinion in Lipidology*, **17**, 631–36.

[3] Shaper, A.G. and Elford, J. (1992) Regional variations in coronary heart disease in Great Britain: risk factors and changes in environment, in *Coronary Heart Disease Epidemiology from Aetiology to Public Health* (eds M. Marmot and P. Elliott), Oxford University Press, New York, pp. 127–39.

[4] Expert Panel on Detection, Evaluation and Treatment of High Blood Cholesterol in Adults (2001) Executive summary of the third report of the National Cholesterol Education Program (NCEP) Expert Panel on Detection, Evaluation, and Treatment of High Blood Cholesterol in Adults (Adult Treatment Panel III). *The Journal of the American Medical Association*, **285**, 2486–97.

[5] Yusuf, S., Hawken, S., Ounpuu, S. *et al.* INTERHEART Study Investigators (2004) Effect of potentially modifiable risk factors associated with myocardial infarction in 52 countries (the INTERHEART study): case-control study. *Lancet*, **364**, 937–52.

[6] Sharrett, A.R., Ballantyne, C.M., Coady, S.A. *et al.* Atherosclerosis Risk in Communities Study Group (2001) Coronary heart disease prediction from lipoprotein cholesterol levels, triglycerides, lipoprotein (a), apolipoproteins A-I and B, and HDL density subfractions: The Atherosclerosis Risk in Communities (ARIC) Study. *Circulation*, **104**, 1108–13.

[7] Carroll, M.D., Lacher, D.A., Sorlie, P.D. *et al.* (2005) Trends in serum lipids and lipoproteins of adults, 1960–2002. *The Journal of the American Medical Association*, **294**, 1773–81.

[8] National Cholesterol Education Program. National Heart, Lung, and Blood Institute. National Institutes of Health. (2002) *Third Report of the National Cholesterol Education Program (NCEP) Expert Panel on Detection, Evaluation, and Treatment of High Blood Cholesterol in Adults (Adult Treatment Panel III)*. Final Report. NIH Publication No. 02-5215. September 2002.

[9] Rosamond, W., Flegal, K., Friday, G. *et al.* The American Heart Association Statistics Committee and Stroke Statistics Subcommittee (2007) Heart Disease and Stroke Statistics – 2007 Update: A Report from the American Heart Association Statistics Committee and Stroke Statistics Subcommittee. http://circ.ahajournals.org/cgi/content/full/115/5/e69. Accessed April 9, 2007.

[10] Law, M.R., Wald, N.J. and Rudnicka, A.R. (2003) Quantifying effect of statins on low density lipoprotein cholesterol, ischaemic heart disease, and stroke: systematic review and meta-analysis. *British Medical Journal*, **326**, 1423–30.

[11] Cholesterol Treatment Trialists' (CTT) Collaborators (2005) Efficacy and safety of cholesterol-lowering treatment: prospective meta-analysis of data from 90 056 participants in 14 randomised trials of statins. *Lancet*, **366**, 1267–78.

[12] Grundy, S.M., Cleeman, J.I., Merz, C.N. *et al.* Coordinating Committee of the National Cholesterol Education Program (2004) Implications of recent clinical trials for the National Cholesterol Education Program Adult Treatment Panel III Guidelines. *Journal of the American College of Cardiology*, **44**, 720–32.

[13] Maki, K.C., Galant, R. and Davidson, M.H. (2005) Non-high-density lipopro-tein cholesterol: the forgotten therapeutic target. *The American Journal of Cardiology*, **96** (suppl 9A), 59K–64K.

[14] Cohen, J.C., Boerwinkle, E., Mosley, T.H. and Hobbs, H.H. Jr (2006) Sequence variations in PCSK9, low LDL, and protection against coronary heart disease. *The New England Journal of Medicine*, **354**, 1264–72.

[15] Cui, Y., Blumenthal, R.S., Flaws, J.A. *et al.* (2001) Non-high-density lipopro-tein cholesterol level as a predictor of cardiovascular disease mortality. *Archives of Internal Medicine*, **161**, 1413–19.

[16] LRC-CPPT Writing Group (1984) The lipid research clinics coronary primary prevention trial results. I. Reduction in incidence of coronary heart disease. *The Journal of the American Medical Association*, **251**, 351–64.

[17] Pearson, T.A., Laurora, I., Chu, H. and Kafonek, S. (2000) The lipid treatment assessment project (L-TAP): a multicenter survey to evaluate the percent-ages of dyslipidemic patients receiving lipid-lowering therapy and achieving low-density lipoprotein cholesterol goals. *Archives of Internal Medicine*, **160**, 459–67.

[18] Davidson, M.H., Maki, K.C., Pearson, T.A. *et al.* (2005) Results of the National Cholesterol Education Program (NCEP) Evaluation ProjecT Utilizing Novel E-Technology (NEPTUNE) II survey and implications for treatment under the recent NCEP Writing Group recommendations. *The American Journal of Car-diology*, **96**, 556–63.

[19] Ansell, B.J., Fonarow, G.C., Maki, K.C. *et al.* NEPTUNE II Steering Committee (2006) Reduced treatment success in lipid management among women with coronary heart disease or risk equivalents: results of a national survey. *American Heart Journal*, **152**, 976–81.

[20] Clark, L.T., Maki, K.C., Galant, R. *et al.* (2006) Ethnic differences in achieve-ment of cholesterol treatment goals. Results from the National Cholesterol Education Program Evaluation Project Utilizing Novel E-Technology II. *Jour-nal of General Internal Medicine*, **21**, 320–26.

2 Vascular Biology and Atherogenesis

Key Points

- *Arteries are highly evolved conduits comprised of multiple cellular and connective tissue layers. Atherogenesis is a diffuse, biochemically and histologically complex disease.*

- *Endothelial dysfunction initiates a series of changes along the vessel wall predisposing to inflammatory cell infiltration, increased thrombotic tendency, and heightened inflammatory tone.*

- *Atherogenesis is driven by a highly orchestrated set of cell types, interleukins, cytokines, reactive oxygen species (ROS), and pro-oxidative enzymes. There is a continuum of disease beginning with the foam cell and progressing to fatty streaks and ultimately to raised atheromatous plaques.*

- *Sudden plaque rupture with overlying thrombus formation is the accepted etiology for acute coronary syndromes (ACS), including unstable angina and acute myocardial infarction (MI). Atheromatous plaque can undergo sudden transitions and rapidly progress from a stable to an unstable condition.*

- *Because the atherothromobotic process involves lipid deposition, endothelial dysfunction, inflammation and hemostasis, numerous targets exist through which lifestyle and pharmacologic interventions may be able to prevent or retard the process and improve clinical outcomes.*

Practical Lipid Management: Concepts and Controversies   Peter P. Toth and Kevin C. Maki
© 2008 John Wiley & Sons, Ltd

2.1 INTRODUCTION

Atherosclerotic disease is highly prevalent throughout the world. Atherosclerosis is a complex disorder, the development of which is dependent on a broad array of histologic, oxidative, inflammatory, and thrombotic influences. Atherosclerosis begins at a young age and its rate of progression is significantly influenced by well-known risk factors, including age, dyslipidemia, hypertension, cigarette smoking, obesity, sedentary lifestyle, and diabetes mellitus. Since the early 1980s, considerable investigation has shown that the control of risk factors through lifestyle modification and pharmacologic intervention slows or even reverses the course of the disease and decreases risk for such complications as myocardial infarction (MI), stroke, claudication and peripheral arterial disease, sudden death, and the need for revascularization via angioplasty or bypass grafting. Early identification and treatment of risk factors is crucial to the long-term prevention of cardiovascular disease given the fact that the number of coexisting risk factors, their severity, and the duration of exposure determine lifetime risk. Consequently, evaluating global cardiovascular risk burden and treating each identified risk factor to established guideline targets is of considerable importance before the onset of clinical signs and symptoms.

Arteries are histologically and biochemically complex, dynamic structures constitutively exposed to proatherogenic influences in the majority of patients. A large number of pathogenic processes are activated in the vasculature during atherogenesis. Atherosclerosis is a diffuse disease, encompasses multiple vascular distributions, and progresses throughout life. Unfortunately, the first acute coronary syndrome or ischemic cerebrovascular accident is fatal in a substantial percentage of cases with no further opportunity to influence the course of disease.

2.2 ARTERIAL STRUCTURE

Arteries are highly evolved conduits for blood and, one of its most important constituents, oxygen. Oxygen must be available in aerobic cells in order to function as a terminal electron acceptor for oxidative phosphorylation. During vasculogenesis, the arterial wall is organized into multiple layers with distinct cellular and connective tissue constituents, including the intima, media, and adventitia. The intima comprises: (i) an endothelial surface, which interfaces with the arterial lumen and (ii) the lamina propria, which contains smooth muscle cells (SMC), fibroblasts, collagen, and intercellular matrix molecules. The media is composed of SMC, which regulate arterial tone by either contracting or relaxing. The media is separated from the intima and adventitia with internal and external elastic membranes. During atherogenesis, SMC in the media can undergo activation, rearrange their actin cytoskeleton and migrate into the intima where they become incorporated into atheromatous plaques. The adventitia is formed from fibroblasts, collagen, and elastin. The *vasa vasora* and the sympathetic and parasympathetic nerve fibers course through the adventitia. The cellular constituents of these various layers interact through complex signaling circuits.

2.3   ENDOTHELIAL CELL FUNCTION AND DYSFUNCTION

Endothelial cells line the luminal surface of blood vessels and serve a variety of highly specialized functions. Endothelial continuity and barrier function is maintained by the formation of tight junctional complexes between cells [1]. The endothelium helps to regulate vascular tone by secreting nitric oxide (NO). NO is formed by endothelial nitric oxide synthase (eNOS) using the amino acid arginine as a substrate. NO formation is stimulated by acetylcholine, substance P, and bradykinin [2]. Once formed, NO diffuses into the media and activates soluble guanylate cyclase, an enzyme that catalyzes the production of cyclic 5'-guanylate monophosphate (cGMP). As cGMP levels increase, smooth muscles relax, resulting in vasodilatation. Endothelial cells produce other vasodilatory substances as well, including prostacyclin (prostaglandin I_2) and endothelium-derived hyperpolarizing factor. The endothelium forms an antithrombotic surface by producing: (i) tissue plasminogen activator (tPA), an enzyme that converts plasminogen to plasmin, which is a thrombolytic enzyme that hydrolyzes fibrin [3] and (ii) thrombomodulin and heparin sulfate, both of which antagonize the activity of thrombin. Prostacyclin and NO have also been shown to inhibit platelet aggregation along the endothelial surface.

When endothelial cells are exposed to elevated levels of atherogenic lipoproteins, high blood pressure, tobacco-derived toxins, or increased serum levels of glucose, they can become dysfunctional [4]. Endothelial cell dysfunction (ECD) is characterized by a number of changes: first, NO production decreases; second, the endothelial surface becomes more prothrombotic because tPA and prostacyclin production decreases and plasminogen activator inhibitor (PAI; an inhibitor of tPA and fibrinolysis) biosynthesis increases; third, the expression of adhesion molecules increases. Adhesion molecules promote the binding and rolling of inflammatory white blood cells, such as monocytes and lymphocytes, along the endothelial surface and include vascular cell adhesion molecule-1 (VCAM-1), intercellular adhesion molecule-1 (ICAM-1), and a variety of selectins [5]. As monocytes bind to the luminal surface of endothelial cells, they can gain access to the subendothelial space by following a gradient of monocyte chemoattractant protein-1 (MCP-1) [6–8] (Figure 2.1). Monocytes can traverse the endothelial barrier by either: (i) diapedesing in between adjacent endothelial cells (paracytosis) or (ii) moving directly through an endothelial cell (transcytosis) [5, 9, 10]. Monocytes taken up into the vessel wall can then take up residence in the subendothelial space and create an inflammatory nidus within the vessel wall.

In addition to promoting vasodilatation, NO is critical to the inhibition of a number of atherogenic mechanisms. NO decreases the adhesion of platelets to endothelium. In addition to promoting thrombus formation, platelets promote intravascular inflammation by functioning as a source of such inflammatory mediators as platelet-derived growth factor, thrombospondin, platelet factor 4, and transforming growth factor-β, among others [11]. NO also inhibits: (i) the migration of SMC from the media into the subendothelial space, an early event in atherogenesis and (ii) intercellular matrix synthesis and deposition [12] (Figure 2.2). Reduced NO production is highly correlated with atherogenesis [13]. Angiotensin II (AII) is an important mediator of hypertension and is produced from angiotensin I (AI) via

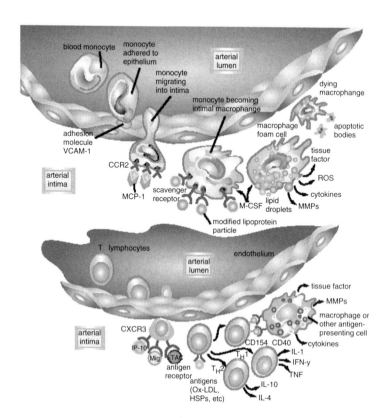

proteolytic hydrolysis by angiotensin converting enzyme (ACE). Dysfunctional endothelium increases its expression of the AT1 receptor, the binding site for AII. Activation of AT1 by AII increases the activity of such enzymes as xanthine oxidase and nicotinamide adenine dinucleotide (phosphate) (NAD(P)H) oxidase [14, 15]. These enzymes increase oxidative stress by increasing the production of ROS, such as superoxide anion, hydroxyl ions, and hydrogen peroxide [16]. The ROS are directly toxic to endothelium, quench NO, and can oxidize and peroxidize the lipids in lipoproteins, thereby rendering them more atherogenic. AII also promotes smooth muscle cell proliferation and migration as well as increased fibroblast collagen production and deposition. Dysfunctional endothelium increases its production of endothelin-1, an extremely potent vasoconstrictor. As endothelium becomes more dysfunctional, gap junctions between cells weaken and the endothelial layer loses functional integrity as a barrier to the

---

Figure 2.1 Inflammatory white cells and atherogenesis. (a) Monocytes in blood can attach to activated endothelial cells by binding to such adhesion molecules as ICAM-1 and VCAM-1. The monocytes can then gain access into the subendothelial space by following a gradient of monocyte chemoattract protein-1 (which binds to the receptor CCR2) and diapedesing across the endothelial cell layer. Once localized to the subendothelial space, the monocytes can transform into macrophages in response to macrophage colony stimulating factor. Macrophages exposed to modified low-density lipoproteins (LDL) express a variety of scavenger receptors that bind and internalize the cholesterol and lipid carried by the LDL particle. As the macrophage becomes progressively more and more loaded with excess cholesterol in the cytosol, it forms lipid inclusion bodies and assumes the histologic characteristics of a "foam cell." Foam cells potentiate inflammation and atherosclerosis by producing matrix metalloproteinases (MMPs), reactive oxygen species such as peroxide and superoxide anion, cytokines, and the procoagulant tissue factor (TF). Foam cells undergo apoptosis (programmed cell death) and necrosis, ultimately facilitating the formation and progression of atheromatous plaques. As enough lipid and cellular debris accumulates, the plaque develops a necrotic core. (b) T lymphocytes or T cells can also infiltrate artery walls after binding to endothelial cell adhesion molecules. T cells follow a gradient of chemoattractants down into the subendothelial space (intima). These chemoattractants bind to the receptor CXCR3 and include monokine-induced by interferon-γ (Mig), inducible protein-10 (IP-10), and interferon-inducible T-cell α-chemoattractant (I-TAC). T cells activated after binding to oxidized LDL or heat shock proteins (HPS) can differentiate further. TH1 cells produce proinflammatory cytokines such as tumor necrosis factor (TNF), interleukin-1 (IL-1), and interferon-γ (IFN-γ). TH2 cells can reduce the intensity of inflammation by producing anti-inflammatory cytokines such as interleukins-4 and 10 (IL-4, IL-10). T cells that express CD154 can interact with CD40 on macrophages and stimulate secretion of TF, MMPs, and other cytokines. Reproduced with permission from Libby, P. (2002) Inflammation in atherosclerosis. *Nature*, **420**, 868–74, [7]. A full-color version of this figure appears in the color plate section of this book.

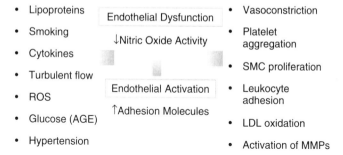

- Lipoproteins
- Smoking
- Cytokines
- Turbulent flow
- ROS
- Glucose (AGE)
- Hypertension

Endothelial Dysfunction
↓Nitric Oxide Activity

Endothelial Activation
↑Adhesion Molecules

- Vasoconstriction
- Platelet aggregation
- SMC proliferation
- Leukocyte adhesion
- LDL oxidation
- Activation of MMPs

Figure 2.2 Factors that induce endothelial cell injury, dysfunction, and activation. Risk factors for cardiovascular disease are injurious to endothelial cells. Endothelial cells exposed to oxidized lipoproteins, increased blood pressure, hyperglycemia, or turbulent blood flow become dysfunctional. Dysfunctional endothelial cells upregulate the expression of adhesion molecules, reactive oxygen species, and PAI-1, and decrease the production of nitric oxide and tPA. This can lead to such proatherogenic changes as increased platelet and white cell adhesion, vasoconstriction, and smooth muscle cell proliferation, among other effects. AGE, advanced glycation end product; LDL, low-density lipoprotein; MMP, matrix metalloproteinase; ROS, reactive oxygen species; SMC, smooth muscle cells. Reproduced with permission from Liao, J. (1998) Endothelium and acute coronary syndromes. *Clinical Chemistry*, **44**, 1799–808, [12].

passage of cells and lipoproteins (i.e. it becomes "leaky"). ECD, as measured by impaired vasoreactivity in response to an acetylcholine or methylcholine challenge [17, 18], and increased expression of PAI-1 are indicators of worse prognosis in patients at risk for cardiovascular events [19]. Endothelial function is improved by increased exercise [20] as well as pharmacologic intervention with statins [21] and ACE inhibitors [22].

2.4 THE ROLE OF MONOCYTES AND LYMPHOCYTES

Monocytes that have become resident in the subendothelial space can undergo a number of histologic transitions (Figure 2.1). When exposed to macrophage colony stimulating factor (M-CSF), the monocyte converts into a macrophage. Macrophages are one of the earliest histologic substrates of atherogenesis. When exposed to oxidatively modified or glycated low-density lipoprotein particles, macrophages upregulate the expression of a number of scavenger receptors on their surface [23]. There are a large number of these scavenger receptors, and include multiple types of scavenger receptor A (types I-III), CD36, lectin-like oxidized low-density lipoproteins receptor-1 (LOX-1), and scavenger receptor for phosphatidyl serine and oxidized low-density lipoproteins (SR-PSOX), among others. These receptors promote the binding and uptake of atherogenic lipoproteins into the intracellular space of the macrophage. As more and more lipid is taken up, the macrophage develops lipid inclusion bodies and becomes a "foam cell." Foam cells produce a variety of cytokines, matrix metalloproteinases (MMPs), ROS, and tissue factor (TF). TF is a procoagulant that promotes platelet aggregation on the surface of ruptured atheromatous plaques [24]. The MMPs can destabilize atheromatous plaques by hydrolyzing the matrix proteins which reinforces their structural integrity. SMC also produce MMPs as they break down the internal elastic lamina in order to access the intima [25]. Ultimately, foam cells can coalesce to form fatty streaks. As fatty streaks increase in volume and more cellular debris accumulates, a frank atheromatous plaque evolves.

T lymphocytes and mast cells also play important roles in atherogenesis. T cells bind to adhesion molecules and can follow a gradient of chemoattractants (inducible protein-10, interferon-inducible T-cell α-chemoattractant, and monokine-induced by interferon-γ) into the subendothelial space [7, 26]. The various chemoattractants can bind to CXCR3, a chemokine receptor on the surface of T cells. When a T cell binds oxidatively modified low-density lipoproteins (LDL) to an antigen receptor it can undergo differentiation into T helper cells, such as TH1 and TH2. TH1 cells potentiate inflammation by producing interleukin-1 (IL-1), interferon-γ, and tumor necrosis factor. TH2 cells can produce anti-inflammatory cytokines, such as interleukin-10. TH1 cells predominate in atheromatous plaques and stimulate inflammation. Following antigen presentation and binding, T cells can stimulate macrophage production of MMPs and cytokines. Activated mast cells are an important source of tryptase and chymase. Chymase catalyzes the conversion of AI to AII within the subendothelial space and tryptase activates the MMPs. Myeloperoxidase, lipoprotein-associated phospholipase A2, cyclooxygenase, and 5'-lipoxygenase are all found in atheromatous plaques and also promote ROS production and oxidative lipoprotein modification [27–29].

2.5 ATHEROMATOUS PLAQUES

During the initial phases of atherogenesis, macrophage foam cells turn into apoptotic bodies and are efficiently cleared by phagocytosis. This orderly clearance process does not promote inflammation. However, as the rate of foam cell formation and accumulation increases, the milieu within the vessel wall changes [30]. More cellular necrosis ensues. The fatty streak progressively enlarges forming an atheromatous plaque with a lipid core and fibrous cap. As an atheromatous plaque evolves, the vessel wall reorganizes in a

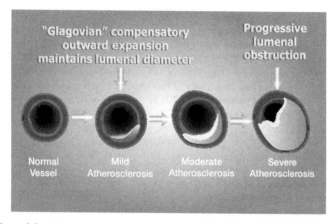

Figure 2.3 Atherosclerosis and vascular remodeling. The traditional depiction of the progression of atherosclerosis entails increasing obstruction of a vessel's lumen. More recent work by Glagov and coworkers suggests a different model. During the early course of atherosclerotic disease, an atheromatous plaque develops outward, in a manner that preserves luminal diameter. This is known as *positive remodeling*. It is only in the later stages of disease that the plaque extends in an intraluminal direction, giving to rise to progressive occlusion and reduced blood flow and ischemia. Reproduced with permission from Nissen, S.H. (2000) Rationale for a postintervention continuum of care: insights from intravascular ultrasound. *The American Journal of Cardiology*, **86**(4B), 12H–17H, [31]. A full-color version of this figure appears in the color plate section of this book.

way that helps to preserve luminal caliber and blood flow (Figure 2.3) [31]. This is known as *positive* or *Glagovian* remodeling [32]. Plaque initially progresses outward, resulting in vessel wall ectasia. It is only in the later stages of atheromatous plaque development that there develops progressive luminal obstruction and, ultimately, physiologically significant reductions in blood flow and oxygen delivery. Within the plaque, cellular necrosis promotes increased inflammation which accelerates atherogenesis and destabilizes plaques [33, 34]. Maintaining the stability of a plaque is tantamount to preventing acute cardiovascular events. Unstable plaques are characterized by large lipid cores, high inflammatory tone (increased macrophage density and increased inflammatory mediator expression), and decreased smooth muscle cell volume [35]. In contrast, stable plaques have increased smooth muscle cell density, low inflammatory tone, small macrophage infiltrates, and a small lipid core. Calcification of plaque also tends to render it more stable. Superficial surface erosions, plaque ulceration, and frank plaque rupture expose the lipid core to blood [34, 36–39]. Tissue factor (TF) and exposed collagen promote platelet degranulation and aggregation, resulting in an overlying thrombus (Figure 2.4). If the thrombus completely

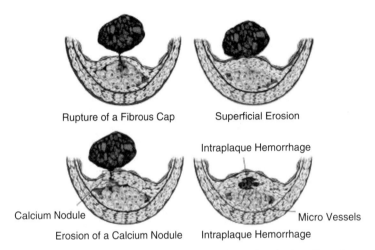

Rupture of a Fibrous Cap   Superficial Erosion

Intraplaque Hemorrhage

Calcium Nodule   Micro Vessels

Erosion of a Calcium Nodule   Intraplaque Hemorrhage

Figure 2.4 Ultrastructural views of atheromatous plaque thrombosis and intraplaque hemorrhage. Scenarios giving rise to architectural disruption of atheromatous plaque and overlying thrombus formation include: rupture of a fibrous cap (upper left), a superficial erosion (upper right), and erosion of a calcific nodule (lower left). When the vasa vasora at the base of an atheromatous plaque leak or are damaged, an intra-plaque hemorrhage can result. This can give rise to sudden increases in plaque pressure and architectural distortion leading to an increase in plaque volume. If the volume of blood entering a plaque is large enough, it can lead to sudden plaque rupture and formation of overlying thrombus. Reproduced with permission from Libby, P. and Theroux, P. (2005) Pathophysiology of coronary artery disease. *Circulation*, **111**, 3481–88, [36].

occludes the arterial lumen, the patient experiences an ST-segment elevating MI (ST-segment elevating myocardial infarction (STEMI)). If thrombus is only partially occluding, the patient experiences unstable angina or a non-ST-segment elevating myocardial infarction (NSTEMI). Patients can experience intermittently recurring chest pain from a single plaque that cyclically forms and lyses thrombus over a smoldering plaque. Inhibitors of platelet aggregation; (aspirin and glycoprotein IIb/IIIa inhibitors) substantially reduce risk for acute coronary syndromes (ACS; including unstable angina and MI). A thin fibrous cap provides less structural reinforcement against plaque fracture and opening in response to a sudden stressor, such as vasospasm or hemorrhaging into the base of a plaque from an injured or leaky *vasa vasora*. Hemorrhaging into the base of a plaque is recognized as an important cause of atheromatous plaque rupture. A sudden rise in the volume of a plaque can lead to loss of architectural integrity. In addition, recurrent hemorrhage into the base of a plaque secondary to leaky *vasa vasora* can lead to repetitive trauma, augmented entry of inflammatory white cells, and increased deposition of cholesterol and lipid in the core of the plaque [40]. As red cells are cleared from the plaque's interior, cholesterol is left behind and functions as a substrate for expansion of the plaque's lipid core. Over time, this too can lead to plaque destabilization.

The plaques that are least likely to rupture are the ones that are calcified and fibrotic. Greater than 80% of all plaque ruptures occur in lesions that are less than 50% obstructive, in part because more of these often exist than larger, more obstructive plaques. Vulnerable lesions (lesions prone to rupture and give rise to ACS) are frequently not identified on coronary angiography, highlighting the importance of primary prevention. There is mounting evidence that aggressive, comprehensive management of risk factors for coronary heart disease (CHD) is associated with significant reductions in risk for ACS and mortality, and that such measures produce plaque stabilization, and, in some instances, plaque regression [41].

REFERENCES

[1] Liebner, S., Cavallaro, U. and Dejana, E. (2006) The multiple languages of endothelial cell-to-cell communication. *Arteriosclerosis, Thrombosis, and Vascular Biology*, **26**, 1431–38.
[2] John, S. and Schmieder, R.E. (2000) Impaired endothelial function in arterial hypertension and hypercholesterolemia: potential mechanisms and differences. *Journal of Hypertension*, **18**, 363–74.
[3] Oliver, J.J., Webb, D.J. and Newby, D.E. (2005) Stimulated tissue plasminogen activator release as a marker of endothelial function in humans. *Arteriosclerosis, Thrombosis, and Vascular Biology*, **5**, 2470–79.
[4] Gibbons, G.H. and Dzau, V.J. (1994) The emerging concept of vascular remodeling. *The New England Journal of Medicine*, **330**, 1431–38.
[5] Rao, R.M., Yang, L., Garcia-Cardena, G. and Luscinskas, F.W. (2007) Endothelial-dependent mechanisms of leukocyte recruitment to the vascular wall. *Circulation Research*, **101**, 234–47.
[6] Libby, P. (2002) Atherosclerosis: the new view. *Scientific American*, **286**, 46–55.
[7] Libby, P. (2002) Inflammation in atherosclerosis. *Nature*, **420**, 868–74.
[8] Libby, P. and Aikawa, M. (2002) Stabilization of atherosclerotic plaques: new mechanisms and clinical targets. *Nature Medicine*, **8**, 1257–62.
[9] Yang, L., Froio, R.M., Sciuto, T.E. *et al.* (2005) ICAM-1 regulates neutrophil adhesion and transcellular migration of TNF-alpha-activated vascular endothelium under flow. *Blood*, **106**, 584–92.
[10] Carman, C.V. and Springer, T. (2004) A transmigratory cup in leukocyte diapedesis both through individual vascular endothelial cells and between them. *The Journal of Cell Biology*, **167**, 377–88.
[11] Libby, P. and Simon, D.I. (2001) Inflammation and thrombosis: the clot thickens. *Circulation*, **103**, 1718–20.
[12] Liao, J.K. (1998) Endothelium and acute coronary syndromes. *Clinical Chemistry*, **44**, 1799–808.

[13] Kuhlencordt, P.J., Gyurko, R., Han, F. *et al*. (2001) Accelerated atherosclerosis, aortic aneurysm formation, and ischemic heart disease in apolipoprotein E/endothelial nitric oxide synthase double-knockout mice. *Circulation*, **104**, 448–54.

[14] Spiekermann, S., Landmesser, U., Dikalov, S. *et al*. (2003) Electron spin resonance characterization of vascular xanthine and NAD(P)H oxidase activity in patients with coronary artery disease: relation to endothelium-dependent vasodilation. *Circulation*, **107**, 1383–89.

[15] Liu, J., Yang, F., Yang, X.P. *et al*. (2003) NAD(P)H oxidase mediates angiotensin II-induced vascular macrophage infiltration and medial hypertrophy. *Arteriosclerosis, Thrombosis, and Vascular Biology*, **23**, 776–82.

[16] Heistad, D.D. (2006) Oxidative stress and vascular disease: 2005 Duff lecture. *Arteriosclerosis, Thrombosis, and Vascular Biology*, **26**, 689–95.

[17] Anderson, T.J., Uehata, A., Gerhard, M.D. *et al*. (1995) Close relation of endothelial function in the human coronary and peripheral circulations. *Journal of the American College of Cardiology*, **26**, 1235–41.

[18] Anderson, T.J., Gerhard, M.D., Meredith, I.T. *et al*. (1995) Systemic nature of endothelial dysfunction in atherosclerosis. *The American Journal of Cardiology*, **75**, 71B–74B.

[19] Sobel, B.E., Woodcock-Mitchell, J., Schneider, D.J. *et al*. (1998) Increased plasminogen activator inhibitor type 1 in coronary artery atherectomy specimens from type 2 diabetic compared with nondiabetic patients: a potential factor predisposing to thrombosis and its persistence. *Circulation*, **97**, 2213–21.

[20] Hambrecht, R., Wolf, A., Gielen, S. *et al*. (2000) Effect of exercise on coronary endothelial function in patients with coronary artery disease. *The New England Journal of Medicine*, **342**, 454–60.

[21] Wassmann, S. and Nickenig, G. (2003) Interrelationship of free oxygen radicals and endothelial dysfunction–modulation by statins. *Endothelium*, **10**, 23–33.

[22] Britten, M.B., Zeiher, A.M. and Schachinger, V. (1999) Clinical importance of coronary endothelial vasodilator dysfunction and therapeutic options. *Journal of Internal Medicine*, **245**, 315–27.

[23] Moore, K.J. and Freeman, M.W. (2006) Scavenger receptors in atherosclerosis: beyond lipid uptake. *Arteriosclerosis, Thrombosis, and Vascular Biology*, **26**, 1702–11.

[24] Bach, R.R. (2006) Tissue factor encryption. *Arteriosclerosis, Thrombosis, and Vascular Biology*, **26**, 456–61.

[25] Bujo, H. and Saito, Y. (2006) Modulation of smooth muscle cell migration by members of the low-density lipoprotein receptor family. *Arteriosclerosis, Thrombosis, and Vascular Biology*, **26**, 1246–52.

[26] Hansson, G.K., Libby, P., Schonbeck, U. and Yan, Z.Q. (2002) Innate and adaptive immunity in the pathogenesis of atherosclerosis. *Circulation Research*, **91**, 281–91.

[27] Nicholls, S.J. and Hazen, S.L. (2005) Myeloperoxidase and cardiovascular disease. *Arteriosclerosis, Thrombosis, and Vascular Biology*, **25**, 1102–11.

[28] Koenig, W., Twardella, D., Brenner, H. and Rothenbacher, D. (2006) Lipoprotein-associated phospholipase A_2 predicts future cardiovascular events in patients with coronary heart disease independently of traditional risk factors, markers of inflammation, renal function, and hemodynamic stress. *Arteriosclerosis, Thrombosis, and Vascular Biology*, **26**, 1586–93.

[29] Leopold, J.A. and Loscalzo, J. (2005) Oxidative enzymopathies and vascular disease. *Arteriosclerosis, Thrombosis, and Vascular Biology*, **25**, 1332–40.

[30] Tabas, I. (2005) Consequences and therapeutic implications of macrophage apoptosis in atherosclerosis: the importance of lesion stage and phagocytic efficiency. *Arteriosclerosis, Thrombosis, and Vascular Biology*, **25**, 2255–64.

[31] Nissen, S.E. (2000) Rationale for a postintervention continuum of care: insights from intravascular ultrasound. *The American Journal of Cardiology*, **86**, 12H–17H.

[32] Glagov, S., Weisenberg, E., Zarins, C.K. *et al.* (1987) Compensatory enlargement of human atherosclerotic coronary arteries. *The New England Journal of Medicine*, **316**, 1371–75.

[33] Libby, P. (2001) What have we learned about the biology of atherosclerosis? The role of inflammation. *The American Journal of Cardiology*, **88**, 3J–6J.

[34] Libby, P. (2001) Current concepts of the pathogenesis of the acute coronary syndromes. *Circulation*, **104**, 365–72.

[35] Davies, M.J., Richardson, P.D., Woolf, N. *et al.* (1993) Risk of thrombosis in human atherosclerotic plaques: role of extracellular lipid, macrophage, and smooth muscle cell content. *British Heart Journal*, **69**, 377–81.

[36] Libby, P. and Theroux, P. (2005) Pathophysiology of coronary artery disease. *Circulation*, **111**, 3481–88.

[37] Libby, P. and Aikawa, M. (2001) Evolution and stabilization of vulnerable atherosclerotic plaques. *Japanese Circulation Journal*, **65**, 473–79.

[38] Libby, P. (1995) Molecular bases of the acute coronary syndromes. *Circulation*, **91**, 2844–50.

[39] Libby, P. (2005) Act local, act global: inflammation and the multiplicity of "vulnerable" coronary plaques. *Journal of the American College of Cardiology*, **45**, 1600–2.

[40] Virmani, R., Kolodgie, F.D., Burke, A.P. *et al.* (2005) Atherosclerotic plaque progression and vulnerability to rupture: angiogenesis as a source of intra-plaque hemorrhage. *Arteriosclerosis, Thrombosis, and Vascular Biology*, **25**, 2054–61.

[41] Boden, W.E., O'Rourke, R.A., Teo, K.K. *et al.* (2007) Optimal medical therapy with or without PCI for stable coronary disease. *The New England Journal of Medicine*, **356**, 1503–16.

3 Detection, Evaluation, and Treatment Goals for Lipid Disorders in Adults

Key Points

- *The National Cholesterol Education Program Adult Treatment Panel (NCEP ATP) III has established three major coronary heart disease (CHD) risk categories with corresponding low-density lipoprotein cholesterol (LDL-C) treatment goals:*

  - *lower risk (0–1 risk factor, LDL-C goal <160 mg dl^{-1});*
  - *moderate risk (2+ risk factors, LDL-C goal <130 mg dl^{-1}); and*
  - *higher risk (CHD or risk equivalent, LDL-C goal <100 mg dl^{-1}).*

- *A three-step process may be used to quickly identify the major CHD risk category:*

  - *Identify CHD or a risk equivalent (diabetes or clinical atherosclerosis), if present, this establishes an LDL-C goal <100 mg dl^{-1}.*
  - *For the remaining patients, major CHD risk factors are counted, if 0–1 major risk factors is present the LDL-C goal is <160 mg dl^{-1}.*
  - *For those not yet classified, the Framingham risk score is calculated in order to determine whether the patient has a 10-year risk $>20\%$ (considered a CHD risk equivalent with an LDL-C goal <100 mg dl^{-1}) or a 10-year CHD risk $\leq20\%$ (LDL-C goal <130 mg dl^{-1}).*

- *Once the major CHD risk category is established, those subsets of patients at very high risk (established cardiovascular disease plus multiple or severe risk factors, optional LDL-C goal <70 mg dl^{-1}) or moderately high risk (10-year event risk 10–20%, optional LDL-C goal*

Practical Lipid Management: Concepts and Controversies   Peter P. Toth and Kevin C. Maki
© 2008 John Wiley & Sons, Ltd

<100 mg dl^{-1}) may be identified for consideration of more aggressive lipid management.

- For patients with high or very high triglycerides ($\geq$200 mg dl^{-1}), non-high-density lipoprotein cholesterol (non-HDL-C) has been established as a secondary target of therapy (after the LDL-C goal has been achieved), with treatment goals that are 30 mg dl^{-1} above the corresponding LDL-C goals.

- No specific treatment goals have been established by the NCEP for triglycerides or HDL-C *per se*, but therapeutic efforts to improve these lipids through lifestyle and drug therapy are encouraged and improvements in these lipids will normally occur as a byproduct of efforts to achieve LDL-C and non-HDL-C treatment goals.

The NCEP Expert Panel on Detection, Evaluation and Treatment of High Blood Cholesterol in Adults (Adult Treatment Panel or ATP) has issued three major sets of clinical guidelines for cholesterol testing and management since 1988, as well as less comprehensive periodic updates as new evidence has accumulated. This chapter is intended to summarize the major recommendations of the ATP III report [1, 2], as well as the 2004 update that established new, more aggressive optional treatment goals for patients at moderately high and very high risk. Specific treatment strategies will not be discussed, as these are covered in Chapters 5–7.

3.1 MATCHING AGGRESSIVENESS OF TREATMENT TO ABSOLUTE RISK

A central feature of all of the ATP reports has been matching the intensity of treatment to the absolute risk for a cardiovascular event. Since events related to CHD (CHD, non-fatal myocardial infarction or coronary death) are the most common types of major cardiovascular events, and the most studied primary outcomes in lipid intervention trials, risk stratification in the ATP III scheme is based on an algorithm designed to classify the patient into major CHD event risk categories. These each have corresponding treatment goals for LDL-C as a primary target, as well as non-HDL-C as a secondary target for patients with elevated triglycerides ($\geq$200 mg dl^{-1}).

3.2 SCREENING FOR DYSLIPIDEMIAS

A screening fasting lipid profile is recommended at least once every five years for all adults $\geq$20 years of age. A fasting lipid profile allows evaluation of total cholesterol, LDL-C (calculated), HDL-C, non-HDL-C, and

Table 3.1 National Cholesterol Education Program Adult Treatment Panel III classification of lipoprotein and total cholesterol and triglyceride levels in adults.

LDL cholesterol (mg dl^{-1})	
<100	Optimal
100–129	Near or above optimal
130–159	Borderline high
160–189	High
≥190	Very high
Total cholesterol (mg dl^{-1})	
<200	Desirable
200–239	Borderline high
≥240	High
HDL cholesterol (mg dl^{-1})	
<40	Low
≥60	High
Triglycerides (mg dl^{-1})	
<150	Normal
150–199	Borderline high
200–499	High
≥500	Very high

From Expert Panel (2001). *The Journal of the American Medical Association*, **285**, 2486–97, [1].

triglyceride concentrations. If the screening lipid profile is nonfasting, it should be followed up with a fasting lipid profile if total cholesterol is ≥200 mg dl^{-1} or the HDL-C level is <40 mg dl^{-1}. Table 3.1 shows the NCEP ATP III classifications for LDL-C, total cholesterol, HDL-C, and triglyceride concentrations.

The total circulating cholesterol level is comprised of cholesterol carried by various lipoproteins. The major lipoproteins are VLDL (very low-density lipoprotein), LDL, and HDL. Normally, the Friedewald equation is used to estimate very low-density lipoprotein cholesterol (VLDL-C) in clinical practice as one-fifth the circulating triglyceride level [3]. In turn, this allows calculation of LDL-C. Thus,

$$LDL\text{-}C = Total\text{-}C - HDL\text{-}C - VLDL\text{-}C$$

This equation can also be stated as follows using the Friedewald formula to estimate the VLDL-C concentration:

$$LDL\text{-}C = Total\text{-}C - HDL\text{-}C - Triglycerides/5$$

The Friedewald equation works well as long as the triglyceride concentration is not >400 mg dl^{-1}. When this is the case, the LDL-C level should be measured directly using either ultracentrifugation or one of several commercially available enzymatic methods. Alternatively, the non-HDL-C level (Total-C minus HDL-C) can be used to guide treatment. Non-HDL-C treatment goals are discussed later in this chapter.

3.3   RISK STRATIFICATION

LDL-C is the primary target for lipid management and the aggressiveness with which it is managed in the ATP III treatment scheme is related to the absolute risk for a CHD event. Therefore, the ATP III has established risk categories with corresponding LDL-C goals. These categories are based on the presence of risk determinants other than LDL-C, including clinical atherosclerosis, diabetes, and major CHD risk factors. Table 3.2 shows the major CHD risk factors. Table 3.3 shows the major CHD risk categories and subcategories, along with the corresponding LDL-C treatment goals.

Table 3.2 Major coronary heart disease risk factors (excluding LDL cholesterol)[a].

Cigarette smoking
Hypertension

- systolic blood pressure ≥ 140 mmHg or diastolic blood pressure ≥ 90 mmHg

- or use of antihypertensive medication

Family history of premature CHD

- CHD in a male first degree relative[b] <55 yr of age

- CHD in a female first degree relative[b] <65 yr of age

Age

- ≥ 45 yr of age for men

- ≥ 55 yr of age for women

HDL cholesterol <40 mg dl^{-1}

- if ≥ 60 mg dl^{-1}, this counts as a "negative risk factor," subtracting 1 from the total

[a] LDL cholesterol is not included among the risk factors because the purpose of counting risk factors is to modify treatment of LDL. Diabetes is a coronary heart disease risk equivalent, so is not counted as a major risk factor in the ATP III classification system.
[b] First degree relatives include parents, siblings, and children.

From Expert Panel (2001) *The Journal of the American Medical Association*, **285**, 2486–97, [1].

Table 3.3   Adult Treatment Panel III risk categories and subcategories with corresponding LDL cholesterol treatment goals.

Risk category	LDL-C goal (mg dl^{-1})
Lower risk: 0–1 risk factor	<160
Moderate risk: ≥2 risk factors[a]	
• 10-yr risk <10%	<130
• 10-yr risk 10–20%	<130, <100 (optional)
High risk: CHD or risk equivalent[b]	
• Other than very high risk	<100
• Very high risk	<100, <70 (optional)

[a] In the absence of CHD or a risk equivalent, 10-yr CHD risk estimates are based on the Framingham risk score.

[b] CHD includes history of myocardial infarction, any evidence of myocardial ischemia, or coronary artery disease. CHD risk equivalents include any form of non-CHD clinical atherosclerosis, multiple risk factors conferring 10-yr CHD risk >20%, or diabetes.

From Expert Panel (2001) *The Journal of the American Medical Association*, **285**, 2486–97, [1].

3.4 STEPS IN THE RISK STRATIFICATION PROCESS – MAJOR RISK CATEGORIES

The following is a practical and somewhat simplified three-step summary of the ATP III risk stratification process. These initial steps are intended to quickly determine the major risk category appropriate for the patient. Once the major risk category is determined, later procedures deal with classifying patients in the 2+ risk factor category into "moderate" and "moderately high" subgroups, as well as classifying those with CHD or risk equivalents into "high" and "very high" risk subgroups.

Step 1. Identify patients with CHD and easily identifiable CHD risk equivalents. Many patients are easy to classify because they have CHD or an easily identifiable CHD risk equivalent and are thus classified into the high risk category (LDL-C goal <100 mg dl^{-1}). Easy to identify CHD risk equivalents include diabetes mellitus (type 1 or type 2) and the presence of non-CHD atherosclerotic disease such as claudication, abdominal aortic aneurysm, or a history of stroke or transient ischemic attack.

Step 2. Count major CHD risk factors in the remaining patients. The next step is to sum the major CHD risk factors shown in Table 3.2. Many patients, particularly younger individuals, will have 0 or 1 major CHD risk factor, and can therefore be classified into the lower risk (LDL-C goal <160 mg dl^{-1}). Because such individuals almost always have 10-year CHD event risk $<10\%$, routine calculation of the Framingham risk score is not required for them.

Step 3. Calculate the Framingham risk score. The remaining patients will be classified as either moderate risk (LDL-C goal <130 mg dl^{-1}) or high risk (LDL-C goal <100 mg dl^{-1}) based on their 10-year probability of a hard CHD event. This is estimated by calculating the Framingham risk score (FRS). The FRS uses information on sex, age, total cholesterol, HDL-C, systolic blood pressure, treatment for hypertension, and cigarette smoking. Points are assigned for each risk factor using the sex-specific values shown in Tables 3.4 and 3.5. The points are then summed and the 10-year CHD event risk corresponding with this sum is assigned based on the values at the bottoms of Tables 3.4 and 3.5. Risk categories and corresponding treatment goals are summarized in Table 3.6.

3.5   TIPS FOR CALCULATING THE FRAMINGHAM RISK SCORE

Informal surveys of clinicians conducted by the authors suggest that relatively few actually calculate the FRS as recommended by the NCEP. Reasons cited include time constraints and the complexity of the formula. Several tools for use with a personal computer or personal digital assistant are available as aids for FRS calculation.

Another factor that is sometimes cited as a difficulty is that the FRS is intended to be calculated based on the pretreatment levels of total and HDL cholesterol. If a patient is a new referral who is already on treatment, or if they have been treated for several years, it may not be clear what values should be used in the calculation. In such cases it may be necessary to estimate the pretreatment values, which can be done quickly with a bit of practice.

Since the total cholesterol values in the scoring system are in 30 mg dl^{-1} bands, it is usually appropriate to add one, two or three bands, depending on the agent and dose that the subject is taking. Three bands may be appropriate if the patient is on a high-efficacy statin (e.g. atorvastatin, rosuvastatin, simvastatin), particularly if the dosage is above the typical starting level. For other drugs and doses, one or two bands would most likely be correct, depending on how close the measured value is to an upper or lower band limit. Our rule of thumb is "when in doubt, add a band." For HDL-C, the bands are in 10 mg dl^{-1} increments. Since most currently available drugs do not increase HDL-C more than about 8 mg dl^{-1}, it is usually appropriate to use the HDL-C value while on treatment, or to use the adjacent band. It should be noted that the methods above provide only rough estimates of

Table 3.4 Framingham risk score calculation for men.

Age	Points	Total cholesterol	Points ages 20–39	Points ages 40–49	Points ages 50–59	Points ages 60–69	Points ages 70+
20–34	−9	<160	0	0	0	0	0
35–39	−4	160–199	4	3	2	1	0
40–44	0	200–239	7	5	3	1	0
45–49	3	240–279	9	6	4	2	1
50–54	6	≥280	11	8	5	3	1
55–59	8	Nonsmoker	0	0	0	0	0
60–64	10	Smoker	8	5	3	1	1
65–69	11	Systolic blood pressure	Points if untreated		Points if treated		
70–74	12						
75–79	13	<120	0		0		
HDL-C		120–129	0		1		
≥60	−1	130–139	1		2		
50–59	0	140–159	1		2		
40–49	1	≥160	2		3		
<40	2						

	Points	Point total	10-yr risk (%)	Point total	10-yr risk (%)	Point total	10-yr risk (%)
Age		≤4	1	10	6	16	25
TC		5	2	11	8	≥17	≥30
HDL-C		6	2	12	10		
Smoking		7	3	13	12		
SBP		8	4	14	16		
Total		9	5	15	20		

TC, total cholesterol; HDL-C, high-density lipoprotein cholesterol.
Total and HDL cholesterol values in milligrams per deciliter, systolic blood pressure in millimeters of mercury.

the effects of treatment on lipid levels for the purpose of risk stratification and are not specifically endorsed by the NCEP.

An alternative method for estimating the pretreatment level of total cholesterol is to use the average percent reduction in cholesterol elicited by the medication (most commonly a statin) and back calculate the pretreatment level. Table 3.7 shows reductions in LDL-C and total cholesterol produced by commonly used doses of statin drugs. A factor of 6% may be used to estimate the influence of lower or higher doses than those shown in the table because each doubling of a statin dose produces roughly a 6% greater LDL-C response and a 5–6% greater total cholesterol response.

Pretreatment total-C = On-treatment total-C

/(1 − average response as a fraction)

Table 3.5 Framingham risk score calculation for women.

Age	Points	Total cholesterol	Points ages 20–39	Points ages 40–49	Points ages 50–59	Points ages 60–69	Points ages 70+
20–34	−7	<160	0	0	0	0	0
35–39	−3	160–199	4	3	2	1	1
40–44	0	200–239	8	6	4	2	1
45–49	3	240–279	11	8	5	3	2
50–54	6	≥280	13	10	7	4	2
55–59	8	Nonsmoker	0	0	0	0	0
60–64	10	Smoker	9	7	4	2	1
65–69	12	Systolic blood pressure	Points if untreated		Points if treated		
70–74	14	<120	0		0		
75–79	16	120–129	1		3		
HDL-C		130–139	2		4		
≥60	−1	140–159	3		5		
50–59	0	≥160	4		6		
40–49	1						
<40	2						

	Points	Point total	10-yr risk (%)	Point total	10-yr risk (%)	Point total	10-yr risk (%)
Age		≤13	≤1	18	6	24	27
TC		13	2	19	8	≥25	≥30
HDL-C		14	2	20	11		
Smoking		15	3	21	14		
SBP		16	4	22	17		
Total		17	5	23	22		

TC, total cholesterol; HDL-C, high-density lipoprotein cholesterol.
Total and HDL cholesterol values in milligrams per deciliter, systolic blood pressure in millimeters of mercury.
From Expert Panel (2001) *The Journal of the American Medical Association*, **285**, 2486–97, [1].

For example, if a patient has a total cholesterol level of 154 mg dl^{-1} while on 40 mg day^{-1} of simvastatin (Zocor), his estimated pretreatment value would be calculated as follows. Table 3.7 shows that the average total cholesterol response to 20 mg day^{-1} of simvastatin is 32%. Because the patient is taking 40 mg day^{-1}, add 6%, producing an estimated effect of 38% or 0.38 when expressed as a fraction. Thus, the estimated pretreatment cholesterol level would be:

$$154 \text{ mg dl}^{-1}/(1 - 0.38) = 248 \text{ mg dl}^{-1}$$

Note that the difference between the estimated pretreatment value and the on-treatment value is 94 mg dl^{-1}, which would translate to an increase of three bands in the FRS calculation (Tables 3.4 and 3.5).

Table 3.6 Adult Treatment Panel III risk categories and subcategories with corresponding LDL cholesterol treatment goals.

Risk category	LDL-C goal (mg dl^{-1})	Non-HDL-C goal (mg dl^{-1})
Lower risk: 0–1 risk factor	<160	<190
Moderate risk: ≥2 risk factors[a]		
• 10-yr risk <10%	<130	<160
• 10-yr risk 10–20%	<130	<160
	<100 (optional)	<130 (optional)
High risk: CHD or risk equivalent[b]		
• Other than very high risk	<100	<130
• Very high risk	<100	<130
	<70 (optional)	<100 (optional)

[a] In the absence of CHD or a risk equivalent, 10-yr CHD risk estimates are based on the Framingham risk score.

[b] CHD includes history of myocardial infarction, any evidence of myocardial ischemia, or coronary artery disease. CHD risk equivalents include any form of non-CHD clinical atherosclerosis, multiple risk factors conferring 10-yr CHD risk >20%, or diabetes.

From Expert Panel (2001) *The Journal of the American Medical Association*, **285**, 2486–2497, [1].

Table 3.7 Effects of commonly used statin doses on levels of low-density lipoprotein cholesterol (LDL-C) and total cholesterol (total-C).

Drug	Dosage (mg d^{-1})	LDL-C reduction $(\%)^a$	Total-C reduction $(\%)^b$
Atorvastatin	10	39	35
Lovastatin	40	31	28
Pravastatin	40	34	31
Simvastatin	20	35	32
Fluvastatin	80	35	32
Rosuvastatin	10	45	41

[a] Estimated LDL-C responses were obtained from US Food and Drug Administration approved package inserts for each product.

[b] Total-C responses were estimated by using a constant of $0.9 \times$ the LDL-C reduction, with all values being rounded to the nearest whole number.

From Expert Panel (2001) *The Journal of the American Medical Association*, **285**, 2486–2497, [1].

3.6 SUBCATEGORIES FOR CONSIDERATION OF MORE AGGRESSIVE OPTIONAL TREATMENT GOALS

Once a patient has been assigned to the lower (0–1 risk factor, LDL-C goal <160 mg dl^{-1}), moderate (2+ risk factors, LDL-C goal <130 mg dl^{-1})

or high (CHD or risk equivalent, LDL-C goal <100 mg dl^{-1}) category, consideration should be given to whether they would be a candidate for more aggressive lipid therapy. The NCEP ATP III established new subcategories with more aggressive optional treatment goals in 2004 [4]. These subcategories are not relevant for patients with 0–1 risk factor.

3.7   VERY HIGH RISK PATIENTS, OPTIONAL LDL-C GOAL <70 mg dl^{-1}

On the basis of evidence from clinical trials suggesting benefits for reducing LDL-C to values well below 100 mg dl^{-1}, the ATP III recommends consideration of an optional LDL-C goal of <70 mg dl^{-1} for patients in the high risk group who have established cardiovascular disease plus any of the following:

1. multiple major risk factors, especially diabetes;
2. severe and/or poorly controlled risk factors, especially smoking;
3. multiple risk factors of the metabolic syndrome, especially triglycerides ≥200 mg dl^{-1}, non-HDL-C ≥130 mg dl^{-1}, HDL-C <40 mg dl^{-1} (non-HDL-C goals are covered later in this chapter and the metabolic syndrome is discussed in Chapter 4);
4. acute coronary syndromes.

3.8   MODERATELY HIGH RISK PATIENTS, OPTIONAL LDL-C GOAL <100 mg dl^{-1}

Based on evidence published since the main ATP III report [1, 2], the NCEP ATP III felt that sufficient evidence had accumulated to recommend consideration of an optional LDL-C goal of <100 mg dl^{-1} for patients whose FRS indicates an estimated 10-year event risk is in the range of 10–20% (moderately high risk).

3.9   TREATMENT GOALS FOR PATIENTS WITH ELEVATED TRIGLYCERIDES

A key theme in the ATP III report is the greater strength of evidence supporting the view that moderate elevations in triglycerides and triglyceride-rich lipoproteins are associated with increased CHD. For patients with very high triglycerides (≥500 mg dl^{-1}), the initial goal of therapy is to lower the triglyceride level to reduce the risk of acute pancreatitis. Regarding CHD risk reduction, achievement of the LDL-C treatment goal is the target for lipid management.

For those with triglycerides ≥ 200 mg dl^{-1}, non-HDL-C goals have also been established as secondary treatment targets. Non-HDL-C goals are each 30 mg dl^{-1} higher than the LDL-C goal for the corresponding risk category (Table 3.6). This is based on the premises that a normal VLDL-C level is ≤ 30 mg dl^{-1} and that the VLDL-C concentration is highly correlated with the concentrations of atherogenic remnant lipoproteins (this is discussed in greater detail in Chapter 6).

3.10   TRIGLYCERIDES AND HDL-C AS TARGETS FOR THERAPY

Although no specific treatment goals have been established by the NCEP for triglycerides or HDL-C *per se*, therapeutic efforts to improve these lipids through lifestyle (low-saturated fat diet, weight loss, and physical activity) and drug therapy are encouraged. Since the available therapies for modification of LDL-C and non-HDL-C levels also typically have favorable effects on triglyceride and HDL-C concentrations, these lipids will generally be improved during the process of achieving the primary (LDL-C) and secondary (non-HDL-C) treatment goals.

CONTROVERSY

SHOULD TREATMENT GUIDELINES INCLUDE TARGETS FOR THE TOTAL/HDL CHOLESTEROL RATIO?

A Proposal for Consideration by the Next Lipid Treatment Guidelines Committee

The Canadian Working Group guidelines for lipid management have advocated treatment goals for the TC/HDL-C ratio, in conjunction with LDL-C (shown in Table 1). Using data from the NEPTUNE II survey, one of the authors assessed the percentages of subjects in each risk category who achieved the NCEP ATP III goals, as well as the percentage who would have achieved the Canadian Working Group goals [1]. Figure 1 shows that a smaller percentage of subjects achieved the Canadian goals, primarily in the CHD and risk equivalents category. This was also true for the subset with high triglycerides (data not shown). Therefore, the addition of TC/HDL-C

Table 1 Canadian Working Group on Hypercholesterolemia and Other Dyslipidemias risk categories and lipid therapy goals.

Risk category	LDL-C goal	TC/HDL-C goal
Low ($\leq$10% 10-yr risk)[a]	<4.5 mmol^{-1} (174 mg dl^{-1})	<6.0
Moderate (11–19% 10-yr risk)[a]	<3.5 mmol^{-1} (135 mg dl^{-1})	<5.0
High ($\geq$20% 10-yr risk)[b]	<2.5 mmol^{-1} (97 mg dl^{-1})	<4.0

[a] 10-yr event risk is calculated with the Framingham Risk Scoring System.

[b] 10-yr event risk is calculated with the Framingham Risk Scoring, but also includes coronary heart disease and risk equivalents.

Adapted from Fodor, J.G. *et al.* (2000) *Canadian Medical Association Journal*, **162**, 1441–47, [2].

targets to the NCEP ATP III LDL-C goals would likely result in more aggressive treatment for those in the highest risk categories. TC/HDL-C goals provide a mechanism through which those with low levels of HDL-C receive more aggressive treatment of atherogenic lipoproteins. The authors suspect that establishment of TC/HDL-C goals for all subjects, without regard to triglyceride level, may prove more effective than the current system, which adds a secondary non-HDL-C goal for patients with hypertriglyceridemia. The TC concentration is less variable day-to-day than the triglyceride level, therefore patients with a slightly elevated triglyceride concentration (e.g. 150–199 mg dl^{-1}), or those who happen to have a lower value when their lipids are checked due to random fluctuations are more likely to receive treatment. For these reasons, as well as others outlined below, the authors favor the establishment of TC/HDL-C goals.

SHOULD THE PRIMARY TARGET FOR THERAPY BE LDL-C OR ATHEROGENIC PARTICLES?

Since the release of the ATP III recommendations, several population and intervention studies have assessed the relative predictive values of LDL-C, non-HDL-C, Apo B, and lipoprotein particle numbers measured with nuclear magnetic resonance. The results have consistently supported the view that the number of atherogenic particles, as indicated by the concentrations of Apo B, non-HDL-C, or VLDL + LDL particles, is a stronger predictor of CHD event risk than the LDL-C concentration [3–6]. In the Framingham and Framingham

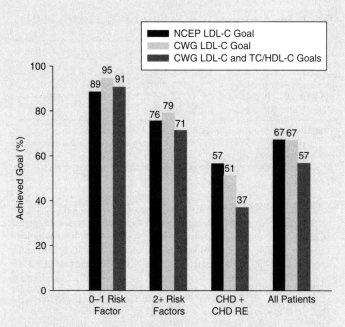

Figure 1 Percentages of 4885 patients who achieved National Cholesterol Education Program (NCEP) and Canadian Working Group (CWG) treatment goals by risk category among participants in a survey of lipid treatment conducted in the United States. LDL-C, low density lipoprotein cholesterol; TC/HDL-C, total cholesterol/high-density lipoprotein cholesterol ratio. Reprinted from Maki, K.C. *et al.* (2006) *The Canadian Journal of Cardiology*, **22**, 315–22, [1].

Offspring cohorts, the relationship between VLDL-C and incident CHD was similar to, and independent of, that for LDL-C among subjects with and without hypertriglyceridemia (Figure 2). Thus, both of the major components of non-HDL-C have independent explanatory value for predicting CHD risk. Moreover, the non-HDL-C level is more strongly correlated with the number of atherogenic particles than LDL-C [3, 7] and changes in non-HDL-C relate more closely to changes in atherogenic particles than changes in LDL-C [8, 9]. Results from intervention trials suggest that reductions in atherogenic particle numbers are more closely related to event reduction than

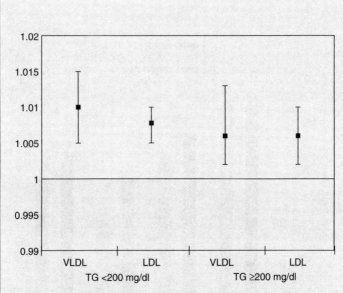

Figure 2 Relative risk for coronary heart disease for each 1 mg dl^{-1} increase in very-low-density lipoprotein (VLDL) and low-density lipoprotein (LDL) cholesterol among participants in the Framingham Heart Study divided into subgroups with and without high triglycerides (TG). Reprinted from Liu, J. *et al.* (2006) *The American Journal of Cardiology*, **98**, 1363–68, [4].

changes in LDL-C among those with and without hypertriglyceridemia [10–14].

The reason that the NCEP ATP III established LDL-C as the primary target for therapy, with non-HDL-C as a secondary target, is the underlying assumption that the LDL-C level is a good proxy for the number of atherogenic particles. However, the results cited above suggest that non-HDL-C is a better indicator of the number of atherogenic particles and therefore a better indicator of CHD event risk. Both the Apo B concentration and the number of atherogenic lipoprotein particles measured with nuclear magnetic resonance may be somewhat better indicators of event risk than non-HDL-C or LDL-C. However, routine use of Apo B or lipoprotein particle concentration measurements is associated with additional cost and complexity. The available data do not provide unequivocal evidence that these are sufficiently more precise indicators of risk to justify the added expense [15]. Non-HDL-C provides a reasonable proxy for the number of atherogenic particles and appears superior to LDL-C, without incremental expense (non-HDL-C is calculated as TC minus HDL-C, so it is available from the lipid profile routinely obtained in clinical settings).

From a practical standpoint, when a patient is treated to a non-HDL-C level less than 30 mg dl^{-1} above their LDL-C goal, the LDL-C concentration is nearly always below the treatment goal. In the NEPTUNE II survey, this was true in >95% of the participants overall and in 100% of the cases for those with triglycerides $\geq$200 mg dl^{-1} (Maki, unpublished observations). In contrast, many patients with LDL-C at goal have non-HDL-C more than 30 mg dl^{-1} above the LDL-C target, and not all of these individuals have triglycerides $\geq$200 mgdl^{-1}. Accordingly, if non-HDL-C goals were simply substituted for LDL-C goals, without regard to triglyceride concentration, it is likely that treatment to goal would result in a greater average reduction in atherogenic particle number than is the case under the NCEP ATP III system.

A Proposal for the Next Treatment Guideline Committee

Based on the currently available evidence, the authors propose that the next lipid guidelines committee give consideration to a scheme like that outlined in Table 2, which contains elements of both the current NCEP ATP III and Canadian Working Group recommendations. The proposed treatment goals have four rather than five risk categories. In the NEPTUNE II survey, 75% of those with CHD and risk equivalents qualified for the very high risk designation. Therefore, for the sake of simplicity, our proposal does not distinguish between the categories of high and very high risk. The moderate risk category encompasses a much larger fraction of the population [16]. Therefore, we have retained the two subgroups. In addition to non-HDL-C goals, we propose including TC/HDL-C targets in order to insure more aggressive treatment of patients with low levels of HDL-C.

Table 2   Proposed treatment goals for consideration by the next National Cholesterol Education Program Adult Treatment Panel.

Risk category	Non-HDL-C goal	TC/HDL-C goal
Lower (0–1 risk factor)	<190 mg dl^{-1}	<4.5
Moderate ($\geq$2 risk factors)		
• 10-yr risk <10%	<160 mg dl^{-1}	<3.5
• 10-yr risk 10–20%	<130 mg dl^{-1}	<3.5
High (CHD or risk equivalent)	<100 mg dl^{-1}	<2.5

Potential Advantages of the Proposed System

We feel that the approach outlined would have several advantages over the current system and other proposed approaches, such as the use of Apo B/Apo AI ratio targets:

1. This approach would require no information beyond that currently provided in the standard lipid profile.
2. In our opinion, this approach is simpler than the current NCEP ATP III recommendations, which include a greater number of risk categories and separate LDL-C and non-HDL-C goals for those with hypetriglyceridemia.
3. Based on data from managed healthcare databases and surveys of clinical practice, the proposed system would likely result in more aggressive treatment of patients at the highest risk, particularly those with low HDL-C and/or high triglycerides. Emerging evidence from clinical trials supports a favorable risk/benefit ratio for more aggressive lipid management in those at high or very high risk.

Potential Disadvantages of the Proposed System

The proposed system is not without possible pitfalls and the main disadvantages are listed below.

1. LDL-C has been designated as the primary target of therapy since the late 1980s and switching would require considerable medical education. Non-HDL-C, although included in the current guidelines, is still unfamiliar to many clinicians and not fully integrated into clinical practice [1].
2. Outcomes trials have not been completed to prospectively investigate the policy of treating to these targets.
3. The available data suggest that measures such as Apo B, the Apo B/Apo AI ratio and concentrations of atherogenic and antiatherogenic lipoprotein particles are somewhat better predictors of CHD risk than non-HDL-C and HDL-C concentrations [3–8]. The main arguments against the use of these alternative measures are that they are more expensive than the standard lipoprotein lipid profile and even more unfamiliar to clinicians than non-HDL-C. If

evidence were to accumulate showing that these approaches have even greater superiority than is evident at present, and/or the cost differential was eliminated for their measurement, consideration would then have to be given to further revisions of the treatment goals.

Many considerations go into the establishment of treatment guidelines, including strength of evidence, cost, ease of implementation, continuity with previous recommendations, etc. Changes in recommendations cannot be undertaken lightly, as compelling arguments can often be advanced for several approaches, each of which will have advantages and disadvantages. Experts reviewing the same evidence frequently reach different conclusions. Therefore, our suggestions are offered not as recommendations for clinicians, but rather as a suggestion for consideration by the next committee writing treatment goals and to stimulate thought and discussion among and between clinicians and scientists.

REFERENCES

[1] Maki, K.C., Davidson, M.H. and Dicklin, M.R. (2006) A comparison of Canadian and American guidelines for lipid management using data from the National Cholesterol Education Program Evaluation ProjecT Utilizing Novel E-technology (NEPTUNE) II survey. *The Canadian Journal of Cardiology*, **22**, 315–22.
[2] Fodor, J.G., Frohlich, J.J., Genest, J.J. Jr and McPherson, P.R. (2000) Recommendations for the management and treatment of dyslipidemia. Report of the Working Group on Hypercholesterolemia and Other Dyslipidemias. *Canadian Medical Association Journal*, **162**, 1441–47.
[3] Cromwell, W.C., Otvos, J.D., Keyes, M.J. *et al.* (2007) LDL particle number and risk of future cardiovascular disease in the Framingham Offspring Study – implications for LDL management. *Journal of Clinical Lipidology*, **1**, 583–92.
[4] Liu, J., Sempos, C.T., Donahue, R.P. *et al.* (2006) Non-high-density lipoprotein and very-low-density lipoprotein cholesterol and their risk predictive values in coronary heart disease. *The American Journal of Cardiology*, **98**, 1363–68.
[5] Ingelsson, E., Schaefer, E.J., Contois, J.H. *et al.* (2007) Clinical utility of different lipid measures for prediction of coronary heart disease in men and women. *The Journal of the American Medical Association*, **298**, 776–85.
[6] Van der Steg, W.A., Boekholdt, S.M., Stein, E.A. *et al.* (2007) Role of the apolipoprotein-B-apoliprotein A-I ratio in cardiovascular risk

assessment: a case-control analysis in EPIC-Norfolk. *Annals of Internal Medicine*, **146**, 640–48.

[7] Grundy, S.M. (2002) Low-density lipoprotein, non-high-density lipoprotein and apolipoprotein B as targets of lipid-lowering therapy. *Circulation*, **106**, 2526–29.

[8] Barter, P.J., Ballantyne, C.M., Carmena, R. *et al.* (2006) Apo B versus cholesterol in estimating cardiovascular risk and in guiding therapy: report of the thirty-person/ten-country panel. *Journal of Internal Medicine*, **259**, 247–58.

[9] Ballantyne, C.M., Andrews, T.C., Hsia, J.A. *et al.* ACCESS Study Group (2001) Atorvastatin Comparative Cholesterol Efficacy and Safety Study. Correlation of non-high-density lipoprotein cholesterol with apolipoprotein B: effect of 5 hydroxymethylglutaryl coenzyme A reductase inhibitors on non-high-density lipoprotein cholesterol levels. *The American Journal of Cardiology*, **88**, 265–69.

[10] Pischon, T., Girman, C.J., Sacks, F.M. *et al.* (2005) Non-high-density lipoprotein cholesterol and apolipoprotein B in the prediction of coronary heart disease in men. *Circulation*, **112**, 3375–83.

[11] Sacks, F.M., Tonkin, A.M., Shepherd, J. *et al.* (2000) Effect of pravastatin on coronary disease events in subgroups defined by coronary risk factors: the Prospective Pravastatin Pooling Project. *Circulation*, **102**, 1893–900.

[12] Farwell, W.R., Sesso, H.D., Buring, J.E. and Gaziano, J.M. (2005) Non-high-density lipoprotein cholesterol versus low-density lipoprotein cholesterol as a risk factor for a first nonfatal myocardial infarction. *The American Journal of Cardiology,* **96**, 1129–34.

[13] Simes, R.J., Marschner, I.C., Hunt, D. *et al.* LIPID Study Investigators (2002) Relationship between lipid levels and clinical outcomes in the Long-term Intervention with Pravastatin in Ischemic Disease (LIPID) Trial: to what extent is the reduction in coronary events with pravastatin explained by on-study lipid levels? *Circulation*, **105**, 1162–69.

[14] Robins, S.J., Collins, D., Wittes, J.T. *et al.* VA-HIT Study Group (2001) Veterans Affairs High-Density Lipoprotein Intervention Trial. Relation of gemfibrozil treatment and lipid levels with major coronary events: VA-HIT: a randomized controlled trial. *The Journal of the American Medical Association*, **285**, 1585–91.

[15] Berkwits, M. and Guallar, E. (2007) Risk factors, risk prediction, and the apolipoprotein B – apolipoprotein A-I ratio. *Annals of Internal Medicine*, **146**, 677–79.

[16] Keevil, J.G., Cullen, M.W., Gangnon, R. *et al.* (2007) Implications of cardiac risk and low-density lipoprotein cholesterol distributions in the United States for the diagnosis and treatment of dyslipidemia: data from National Health and Nutrition Examination Survey 1999 to 2002. *Circulation*, **115**, 1363–70.

REFERENCES

[1] Expert Panel on Detection, Evaluation and Treatment of High Blood Cholesterol in Adults (2001) Executive summary of the third report of the National Cholesterol Education Program (NCEP) Expert Panel on Detection, Evaluation, and Treatment of High Blood Cholesterol in Adults (Adult Treatment Panel III). *The Journal of the American Medical Association,* **285**, 2486–97.

[2] National Cholesterol Education Program. National Heart, Lung, and Blood Institute. National Institutes of Health (2002) Third Report of the National Cholesterol Education Program (NCEP) Expert Panel on Detection, Evaluation, and Treatment of High Blood Cholesterol in Adults (Adult Treatment Panel III). Final Report. *NIH Publication No. 02-5215*, September 2002.

[3] Friedewald, W.T., Levy, R.I. and Fredrickson, D.S. (1972) Estimation of the concentration of low-density lipoprotein cholesterol in plasma, without use of the preparative ultracentrifuge. *Clinical Chemistry*, **18**, 499–502.

[4] Grundy, S.M., Cleeman, J.I., Merz, C.N. *et al.* Coordinating Committee of the National Cholesterol Education Program (2004) Implications of recent clinical trials for the National Cholesterol Education Program Adult Treatment Panel III Guidelines. *Journal of the American College of Cardiology*, **44**, 720–32.

4 Therapeutic Lifestyle Changes in the Management of Lipid Disorders and the Metabolic Syndrome

Key Points

- *A western lifestyle characterized by low physical activity, a diet high in saturated fats and cholesterol, excess energy consumption and a substantial prevalence of cigarette smoking is associated with the development of numerous coronary heart disease (CHD) risk factors, including dyslipidemias, hypertension, obesity, diabetes, and inflammatory and hypercoagulable states.*

- *The metabolic syndrome (MetS) is a cluster of risk factors for CHD and type 2 diabetes that includes: central obesity, elevated triglycerides, reduced high-density lipoprotein cholesterol (HDL-C), elevated blood pressure, and elevated glucose. The prevalence of the MetS is high in the general US population and exceeds 50% among patients undergoing treatment for dyslipidemia.*

- *The National Cholesterol Education Program Adult Treatment Panel (NCEP ATP) III recommends therapeutic lifestyle changes (TLC) as the first line of therapy in the management of dyslipidemias. The primary target of TLC is to reduce low-density lipoprotein cholesterol (LDL-C) to the target level. Secondary targets include achieving non-HDL-C goals and improvements in the components of the MetS. The main features of the TLC recommendations include:*

Practical Lipid Management: Concepts and Controversies   Peter P. Toth and Kevin C. Maki
© 2008 John Wiley & Sons, Ltd

- *reduced intakes of saturated fats (<7% of energy) and cholesterol (<200 mg day^{-1});*
- *dietary adjuncts for lowering LDL-C, including plant sterols/ stanols (2 g day^{-1}) and increased intake of viscous fibers (10–25 g day^{-1});*
- *weight reduction if overweight or obese;*
- *increased physical activity.*

- *Efforts at lifestyle modification often receive less attention than they should in clinical practice. Clinicians are encouraged to employ greater efforts toward TLC in their practices and to utilize nurses, dietitians, and other allied health professionals more frequently to aid patients in achieving clinically important lifestyle modifications.*

As discussed in detail in Chapter 1, potentially modifiable risk factors account for at least 90% of the population attributable risk for CHD. The incidence and prevalence of many of these risk factors are markedly lower in countries where a traditional lifestyle is still prevalent. Moreover, in western countries, the CHD risk factor profile of those with low-risk lifestyle habits is markedly better than that of the general population [1–3]. Thus, variation between and within countries in CHD risk factors can be largely accounted for by variations in lifestyle factors such as diet, physical activity, and cigarette smoking, which lead to the development of metabolic disturbances (obesity, dyslipidemia, hypertension, inflammation, glucose intolerance). Unfortunately, once present, many of these conditions are difficult to reverse and must be managed through a combination of lifestyle changes and drug therapies.

4.1 NATURE AND NURTURE IN THE DEVELOPMENT OF CHD RISK FACTORS

The Pima Indians provide a dramatic illustration of the importance of lifestyle in the development of CHD risk factors. The Pimas who live in Arizona, USA are well known for their exceptionally high rates of obesity and diabetes. By age 35, more than 85% of male Pimas in this region are obese and more than half have type 2 diabetes [4]. In contrast, among Pima Indians living in rural Mexico, who have more traditional lifestyle patterns, obesity and diabetes are markedly less common [4, 5]. This group typically engages in much more physical activity than the Pimas in Arizona and they consume a diet that is low in saturated fats and cholesterol, high in whole grains and legumes, and low in processed grains. While the Pimas in rural Mexico undoubtedly have strong genetic potential for obesity and diabetes, their traditional lifestyle appears to prevent the expression of these traits.

4.2 LIFESTYLE FACTORS AS DETERMINANTS OF CHD RISK IN POPULATIONS

Migration studies have shown that when people move to western countries and adopt western lifestyle patterns, this relocation is followed by increases in the prevalence of CHD risk factors, including hypercholesterolemia, hypertension, obesity, physical inactivity, and diabetes [6, 7]. As might be expected, CHD incidence increases in tandem and is similar to that of the adopted country within one to two generations. A similar pattern is observed as countries adopt more western lifestyle habits. For example, in the Seven Countries Study, the average LDL-C concentration among citizens of Japan in the 1950s was <100 mg dl^{-1}. In contrast, the average total cholesterol level in the USA at that time was >160 mg dl^{-1} [8]. Since that time the influence of western culture on the Japanese lifestyle has increased and the average level of LDL-C has risen. In the USA, the average LDL-C level has declined, in part due to public health efforts aimed at lowering population intakes of saturated fats, *trans* fats, and cholesterol, as well as increases in the use of cholesterol-lowering medications [9, 10]. Thus, the changes in lifestyle (and other factors) in the populations have resulted in the two countries having very similar average LDL-C concentrations ($\sim$130 mg dl^{-1}) early in the twenty-first century [11].

4.3 WITHIN COUNTRY VARIATIONS IN LIFESTYLE AND CHD RISK

Within the USA and other western countries, people who maintain lifestyle habits similar to those recommended in national guidelines are less likely to have major CHD risk factors and show lower incidence rates for CHD events. For example, in the US Nurses' Health Study, female nurses with a low-risk lifestyle pattern had an incidence of major coronary events that was 83% below that of the remainder of the cohort [2]. The low-risk lifestyle pattern included abstinence from cigarette smoking, body mass index <25 kg m^{-2}, at least 30 min day^{-1} of physical activity, moderate alcohol consumption, and a composite dietary score in the top 40% of the population.

  One of the authors of this book was involved in a survey of physicians in suburban Chicago (USA) that assessed the prevalence of being overweight and obese. Only 8% of the participating physicians were obese [12], compared with a prevalence of nearly 35% in the general population [13].

Data from the US Physicians' Health Study show that the incidence of CHD among US male physicians is ~85% lower than that of men in the general population [14]. The lower incidence of CHD can be largely explained by lifestyle habits that are more closely aligned with national recommendations, as well as greater attention to management of major CHD risk factors. Thus, physicians are a model for the potential impact of a low-risk lifestyle and risk factor management on CHD event rates.

4.4 THE METABOLIC SYNDROME

The MetS is a cluster of risk factors for both CHD and type 2 diabetes mellitus that are found together in the same individual more frequently than would be predicted by chance. An impaired ability of insulin to promote cellular uptake of glucose (insulin resistance) is a central pathogenic feature of this syndrome. Insulin resistance is frequently, but not always, associated with excess adiposity, particularly increased levels of abdominal fat. The NCEP ATP III provided a set of criteria for identifying the MetS in clinical practice. These have been subsequently updated and revised in a joint statement from the American Heart Association and the National Heart Lung and Blood Institute [15]. The MetS is diagnosed when at least three of five MetS component risk factors are present (Table 4.1). It should be noted that the clinical definition of the MetS was selected based on variables that are practical to measure in a clinical setting. However, among those with the MetS, several additional metabolic disturbances are often present, including elevated levels of C-reactive protein, fibrinogen, uric acid, and insulin.

The estimated age-adjusted prevalence of the MetS in the USA was recently reported to be 27% [16]. The prevalence of the MetS increases dramatically with age, affecting nearly 50% of the population over 60 years [16]. Moreover, the MetS appears to be quite common among patients undergoing treatment for dyslipidemias. In the NEPTUNE II survey of subjects receiving outpatient lipid management, the prevalence of the MetS was 62% overall and 74% among patients with CHD or CHD risk equivalents (including diabetes) [17].

Lifestyle plays a central role in the development of the MetS. Since 1980, the prevalence of obesity in the USA has more than doubled. The percentage of the population who are overweight or obese, as indicated by body mass index ≥ 25 kg m^{-2}, exceeds 65% [13, 18]. During this same period, physical activity among children and adults has declined steadily [13]. Both of these changes have contributed substantially to the high prevalence of the MetS in the US population, including an alarming prevalence among children and adolescents [19]. The NCEP ATP III has identified the MetS risk factors as a secondary target for intervention after achievement of LDL-C treatment goals.

Table 4.1 Criteria for clinical diagnosis of metabolic syndrome.

Measure (any 3 of 5 constitute diagnosis of metabolic syndrome)	Categorical cutpoints
Elevated waist circumference[a,b]	$\geq$102 cm in men $\geq$88 cm in women
Elevated triglycerides	$\geq$150 mg dl^{-1} (1.7 mmol l^{-1}) **Or** On drug treatment for elevated triglycerides[c]
Reduced HDL-C	<40 mg dl^{-1} (0.9 mmol l^{-1}) in men <50 mg dl^{-1} (1.1 mmol l^{-1}) in women **Or** On drug treatment for reduced HDL-C[c]
Elevated blood pressure	$\geq$130 mmHg systolic blood pressure **Or** $\geq$85 mmHg diastolic blood pressure **Or** On antihypertensive drug treatment in a patient with a history of hypertension
Elevated fasting glucose	$\geq$100 mg dl^{-1} **Or** On drug treatment for elevated glucose

[a] To measure waist circumference, locate top of right iliac crest. Place a measuring tape in a horizontal plane around abdomen at level of iliac crest. Before reading the tape measure, ensure that tape is snug but does not compress the skin and is parallel to floor. Measurement is made at the end of a normal expiration.

[b] Some US adults of non-Asian origin (e.g. White, Black, Hispanic) with marginally increased waist circumference (e.g. 94–102 cm (37–39 in.) in men and 80–88 cm (31–35 in.) in women) may have strong genetic contribution to insulin resistance and should benefit from changes in lifestyle habits, similar to men with categorical increases in waist circumference. Lower waist circumference cutpoint (e.g. $\geq$90 cm (35 in.) in men and $\geq$80 cm (31 in.) in women) appears to be appropriate for Asian Americans.

[c] Fibrates and nicotinic acid are the most commonly used drugs for elevated TG and reduced HDL-C. Patients taking one of these drugs are presumed to have high TG and low HDL.

From Grundy *et al.* (2005) *Circulation*, **112**, e285–90, [15] with kind permission of Lippincott Williams & Wilkins.

4.5   THERAPEUTIC LIFESTYLE CHANGES

The NCEP ATP III recommends TLC as the first line of therapy for patients with dyslipidemia (Figure 4.1). The guidelines recommend that lifestyle changes should be given an adequate trial (three to six months) before

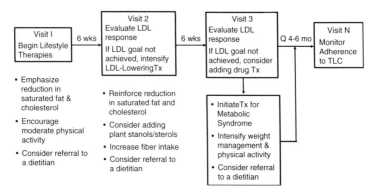

Figure 4.1 A model of steps in therapeutic lifestyle Changes (TLC). From Expert Panel (2001) *The Journal of the American Medical Association*, **285**, 2486–97, [20].

institution of drug therapy, although for patients with CHD or risk equivalents, consideration may be given to instituting drug therapy and TLC simultaneously, particularly for those with LDL-C levels substantially above goal. The primary target of TLC is to lower the LDL-C level to the treatment goal for the patient's risk category. Secondary targets after achievement of the LDL-C goal are to reduce non-HDL-C to the treatment goal and to improve triglyceride and HDL-C concentrations.

The main features of the TLC recommendations include:

- reduced intakes of saturated fats (<7% of energy) and cholesterol (<200 mg day^{-1});

- dietary adjuncts for lowering LDL-C, including plant sterols/stanols (2 g day^{-1}) and increased intake of viscous fibers (10–25 g day^{-1});

- weight reduction if overweight or obese;

- increased physical activity.

4.6 THE TLC DIET

Recommendations for the nutrient composition of the TLC diet are shown in Table 4.2 [20]. Compared to previous dietary recommendations from the NCEP, the TLC diet has greater initial emphasis on reducing intakes of saturated fat and cholesterol and less on restriction of total fat intake.

Table 4.2 Nutrient composition of the therapeutic lifestyle changes (TLC) diet.

Nutrient	Recommended intake
Saturated fat[a]	<7% of total calories
Polyunsaturated fat	Up to 10% of total calories
Monounsaturated fat	Up to 20% of total calories
Total fat	25–35% of total calories
Carbohydrate[b]	50–60% of total calories
Fiber	20–30 g day^{-1}
Protein	Approximately 15% of total calories
Cholesterol	<200 mg day^{-1}
Total calories (energy)[c]	Balance energy intake and expenditure to maintain desirable body weight/prevent weight gain

[a] Trans fatty acids are another LDL-raising fat that should be kept at a low intake.
[b] Carbohydrate should be derived predominantly from foods rich in complex carbohydrates including grains, especially whole grains, fruits, and vegetables.
[c] Daily energy expenditure should include at least moderate physical activity (contributing approximately 200 kcal day^{-1}).

From Expert Panel (2001) *The Journal of the American Medical Association*, **285**, 2486–97, [20].

The primary target of lipid management in the NCEP ATP III is lowering LDL-C to the treatment target. Greater intakes of saturated fats and cholesterol fats raise the LDL-C concentration, so restricting the intakes of these dietary components to <7% of energy and <200 mg day^{-1}, respectively, is strongly encouraged. *Trans* fats, such as those found in shortenings and stick margarines also raise LDL-C. While no specific recommendation is made regarding percentage of caloric intake from *trans* fats, it is recommended that their intake be kept as low as possible.

Increased consumption of unsaturated fats (mono- and polyunsaturated) lowers the LDL-C concentration. Furthermore, high dietary carbohydrate content has been associated with increases in triglycerides and very-low-density lipoprotein cholesterol (VLDL-C), as well as reductions in HDL-C. This is especially true for patients with obesity or the MetS [21]. Accordingly, whereas previous recommendations emphasized replacing saturated fats with carbohydrates, the TLC diet recommends replacing saturated fats with a combination of unsaturated fats (e.g. from nuts and liquid oils) and complex carbohydrates, preferably from sources such as whole grains, vegetables, and fruits that also contain dietary fiber. Table 4.3 shows a summary of a low-risk dietary pattern that is consistent with the NCEP ATP III recommendations [1, 3].

Table 4.3 Characteristics of a low-risk dietary pattern consistent with the National Cholesterol Education Program therapeutic lifestyle changes diet.

Foods to be emphasized	Foods to be eaten sparingly
Whole grains	Refined grains
Legumes	White rice and potatoes
Nuts and oils	Stick margarines and shortenings
Fruits and vegetables	Sodas, sweets, and desserts
Fish and lean meats	High-fat meats
Low-fat dairy products	High-fat dairy products

From Maki. (2004) *The American Journal of Cardiology*, **93** (Suppl 11A), 12C–17C, [1].

4.7 DIETARY ADJUNCTS: VISCOUS FIBERS AND PLANT STEROL/STANOL PRODUCTS

If the TLC diet alone is not sufficient to lower LDL-C to the target level, the NCEP ATP III recommends inclusion of dietary sources of viscous fibers (10–25 g day^{-1}) and plant sterol/stanol products (2 g day^{-1} of sterol/stanol) in the diet. In the authors' experience, such recommendations are rarely made in clinical practice. This is unfortunate, since numerous studies have shown that the effects of dietary interventions are additive to those of drug therapies [22–24]. Moreover, each nondrug intervention provides 5–10% reductions in LDL-C, which approximates the degree of LDL-C reduction achieved through doubling the dose of a statin drug [21].

If a patient on a typical American diet (i) reduces their intakes of saturated fat and cholesterol, (ii) adds a rich source of viscous fiber to the diet, and (iii) consumes 2 g day^{-1} of plant sterol, or stanols, the expected reduction in LDL-C would be 15–24%. Additional LDL-C lowering might be achieved by loss of 5–10% of body weight if the patient is overweight or obese. Thus, it is possible to obtain reductions of up to 30% in LDL-C with aggressive dietary and lifestyle management [25–27], although smaller reductions (5–15%) are more commonly achieved in clinical practice.

Examples of good dietary sources of viscous fibers include whole oats and barley, certain fruits such as prunes and pears, and some bulk fiber laxatives including Metamucil and Citrucel. Several plant sterol and/or stanol-containing products are available in grocery stores including margarine-like spreads, yogurts, snack bars, and dietary supplements.

4.8 PHYSICAL ACTIVITY AND WEIGHT REDUCTION

The current recommendations regarding physical activity are for all Americans to engage in 30–60 min of activity on most days or ~1000 kcal per week [26]. Walking is the most practical form of exercise for most people and the average middle-aged man or woman can walk approximately 2 miles in 30 min. A useful rule of thumb is that the number of kcal required to walk a mile is approximately equal to 0.67 times body weight in pounds. Thus, a 150-pound woman will burn about 100 kcal for each mile walked. The corresponding number for a 200-pound man would be 134 kcal.

Increased physical activity and weight loss have independent and additive beneficial effects on numerous CHD risk factors, particularly those of the MetS, including blood pressure, insulin resistance, glucose tolerance, lipid concentrations (mainly triglyceride and HDL-C levels), and markers of inflammation and hemostatic balance. In addition, regular physical activity is extremely important for weight management. It is not necessary to achieve ideal body weight in order for weight loss to have an important impact on the CHD risk factor profile. Clinically important improvements are evident after loss of as little as 5% of body weight.

4.9 SMOKING CESSATION

In addition to being a major CHD risk factor itself, cigarette smoking is associated with adverse changes in numerous CHD risk markers, including levels of triglycerides, HDL-C, insulin resistance, fibrinogen, and other hemostatic and inflammatory markers. For patients who smoke, clinicians should strongly encourage them to quit. For patients who are unwilling or unable to do so, efforts to limit smoking should be encouraged and the significance of managing lipids and other CHD risk factors is heightened.

4.10 IMPORTANCE OF ALLIED HEALTH PROFESSIONALS

The sad truth is that, despite the large potential for TLC to reduce CHD risk, they often receive minimal attention in practice. In part this may reflect nihilism among clinicians who become frustrated with minimal improvements observed after recommending lifestyle changes to many patients. In part it may reflect the fact that time constraints make it very difficult to counsel patients effectively on how to implement lifestyle changes.

Allied health professionals can play an important role in guiding and encouraging patients to undertake lifestyle changes. Nurses, dietitians, exercise physiologists, and social workers can all contribute importantly to the process of behavior change in both primary and secondary prevention. Phases II and III cardiac rehabilitation programs frequently employ some or all of these professionals, who have the time and expertise required to assist patients with implementation of the TLC recommendations. In addition, some managed care organizations and health clubs offer these services. Expense and lack of insurance coverage for such services can be a significant barrier to their use. Therefore, the primary responsibility for learning about and implementing TLC falls to the patient and it is imperative that clinicians counsel patients on the importance of lifestyle in the development and management of cardiovascular risk.

REFERENCES

[1] Maki, K.C. (2004) Dietary factors in the prevention of diabetes mellitus and coronary artery disease associated with the metabolic syndrome. *The American Journal of Cardiology*, **93** (Suppl 11A), 12C–17C.
[2] Stampfer, M.J., Hu, F.B., Manson, J.E. *et al.* (2000) Primary prevention of coronary heart disease in women through diet and lifestyle. *The New England Journal of Medicine*, **343**, 16–22.
[3] Hu, F.B. (2002) Dietary pattern analysis: a new direction in nutritional epidemiology. *Current Opinion in Lipidology*, **13**, 3–9.
[4] Ravussin, E., Valencia, M.E., Esparza, J. *et al.* (1994) Effects of a traditional lifestyle on obesity in Pima Indians. *Diabetes Care*, **17**, 1067–74.
[5] Schultz, L.O., Bennett, P.H., Ravussin, E. *et al.* (2006) Effects of traditional and western environments on prevalence of type 2 diabetes in Pima Indians in Mexico and the US. *Diabetes Care*, **29**, 1866–71.
[6] Shaper, A.G. and Elford, J. (1992) Regional variations in coronary heart disease in Great Britain: risk factors and changes in environment, in *Coronary Heart Disease Epidemiology from Aetiology to Public Health* (eds M. Marmot and P. Elliott), Oxford University Press, New York, pp. 127–39.
[7] Epstein, F.H. (1992) Contribution of epidemiology to understanding coronary heart disease, in *Coronary Heart Disease Epidemiology from Aetiology to Public Health* (eds M. Marmot and P. Elliott), Oxford University Press, New York, pp. 20–32.
[8] Brown, B.G., Stukovsky, K.H. and Zhao, X.Q. (2006) Simultaneous low-density lipoprotein-C lowering and high-density lipoprotein-C elevation for optimum cardiovascular disease prevention with various drug classes, and their combinations: a meta-analysis of 23 randomized lipid trials. *Current Opinion in Lipidology*, **17**, 631–36.
[9] Carroll, M.D., Lacher, D.A., Sorlie, P.D. *et al.* (2005) Trends in serum lipids and lipoproteins of adults, 1960–2002. *The Journal of the American Medical Association*, **294**, 1773–81.

[10] Keevil, J.G., Cullen, M.W., Gangnon, R. *et al.* (2007) Implications of cardiac risk and low-density lipoprotein cholesterol distributions in the United States for the diagnosis and treatment of dyslipidemia: data from National Health and Nutrition Examination Survey 1999 to 2002. *Circulation*, **115**, 1363–70.

[11] Kita, T. (2004) Coronary heart disease risk in Japan – an East/West divide? *European Heart Journal*, **6**, A8–A11.

[12] LaPuma, J., Szapary, P. and Maki, K.C. (2005) Predictors of physician overweight and obesity in the USA: an empiric analysis. *Nutrition and Food Science*, **35**, 315–19.

[13] Manson, J.E., Skerrett, P.J., Greenland, P. and VanItallie, T.B. (2004) The escalating pandemics of obesity and sedentary lifestyle: a call to action for clinicians. *Archives of Internal Medicine*, **164**, 249–58.

[14] Physicians' Health Study Steering Committee (1989) Final report on the aspirin component of the ongoing Physicians' Health Study. *The New England Journal of Medicine*, **321**, 129–35.

[15] Grundy, S.M., Cleeman, J.I., Daniels, S.R. *et al.* (2005) Diagnosis and management of the metabolic syndrome: an American Heart Association/National Heart, Lung, and Blood Institute Scientific Statement. *Circulation*, **112**, e285–90.

[16] Ford, E.S., Giles, W.H. and Mokdad, A.H. (2004) Increasing prevalence of the metabolic syndrome among U.S. adults. *Diabetes Care*, **27**, 2444–49.

[17] Deedwania, P.C., Maki, K.C., Dicklin, M.R. *et al.* (2006) Application of recent definitions of the metabolic syndrome to survey data from the National Cholesterol Education Program Evaluation Project Utilizing Novel E-Technology (NEPTUNE II). *Journal of the Cardiometabolic Syndrome*, **1**, 295–300.

[18] Flegal, K.M., Carroll, M.D., Ogden, C.L. and Johnson, C.L. (2002) Prevalence and trends in obesity among US adults, 1999–2000. *The Journal of the American Medical Association*, **288**, 1723–27.

[19] Weiss, R., Dziura, J., Burgert, T.S. *et al.* (2004) Obesity and the metabolic syndrome in children and adolescents. *The New England Journal of Medicine*, **350**, 2362–74.

[20] Expert Panel on Detection, Evaluation and Treatment of High Blood Cholesterol in Adults (2001) Executive summary of the third report of the National Cholesterol Education Program (NCEP) Expert Panel on Detection, Evaluation, and Treatment of High Blood Cholesterol in Adults (Adult Treatment Panel III). *The Journal of the American Medical Association*, **285**, 2486–97.

[21] Maki, K.C., Galant, R. and Davidson, M.H. (2005) Non-high-density lipoprotein cholesterol: the forgotten therapeutic target. *The American Journal of Cardiology*, **96** (Suppl 9A), 59K–64K.

[22] Katan, M.B., Grundy, S.M., Jones, P. *et al.* Stresa Workshop Participants (2003) Efficacy and safety of plant stanols and sterols in the management of blood cholesterol levels. *Mayo Clinic Proceedings*, **78**, 965–78.

[23] Moreyra, A.E., Wilson, A.C. and Koraym, A. (2005) Effect of combining psyllium fiber with simvastatin in lowering cholesterol. *Archives of Internal Medicine*, **165**, 1161–66.

[24] Goldberg, A.C., Ostlund, R.E., Bateman, J.H. *et al.* (2006) Effect of plant stanol tablets on low-density lipoprotein cholesterol lowering in patients on statin drugs. *The American Journal of Cardiology*, **97**, 376–79.

[25] Maki, K.C., Davidson, M.H. and Dicklin, M.R. (2006) A comparison of Canadian and American guidelines for lipid management using data from the National Cholesterol Education Program Evaluation Project Utilizing Novel E-Technology (NEPTUNE) II survey. *The Canadian Journal of Cardiology*, **22**, 315–22.

[26] National Cholesterol Education Program, National Heart, Lung, and Blood Institute, National Institutes of Health (2002) *Third Report of the National Cholesterol Education Program (NCEP) Expert Panel on Detection, Evaluation, and Treatment of High Blood Cholesterol in Adults (Adult Treatment Panel III)*, Final Report, NIH Publication No. 02-5215.

[27] Jenkins, D.J., Kendall, C.W., Marchie, A. *et al.* (2003) Effects of a dietary portfolio of cholesterol-lowering foods vs lovastatin on serum lipids and C-reactive protein. *The Journal of the American Medical Association*, **290**, 502–10.

5 Management of Elevated Low-density Lipoprotein Cholesterol

Key Points

- *Studies show a clear relationship between low-density lipoprotein cholesterol (LDL-C) and risk for coronary heart disease (CHD), myocardial infarction (MI), peripheral arterial disease, carotid artery disease, ischemic stroke, and sudden death.*

- *Several genetic disorders cause elevated LDL-C, including familial hypercholesterolemia (FH), familial combined hyperlipidemia (FCH), familial defective apolipoprotein B, and autosomal dominant hypercholesterolemia.*

- *The National Cholesterol Education Program Adult Treatment Panel (NCEP ATP III) added an optional treatment goal of <70 mg dl^{-1} for patients at very high-risk, defined as those with established atherosclerotic cardiovascular disease (CVD) plus any of the following: multiple risk factors; severe, poorly controlled risk factors; metabolic syndrome, diabetes mellitus or a history of acute coronary syndromes (MI or unstable angina). Results from clinical trials have supported the view that lowering LDL-C levels to values well below 100 mg dl^{-1} has incremental benefit in very high-risk subgroups.*

- *The management of elevated LDL-C is focused on instituting therapeutic lifestyle changes (TLC), followed by pharmacologic therapy (mainly statins, ezetemibe, bile acid sequestrants (BASs)) if necessary to achieve LDL-C treatment targets.*

Practical Lipid Management: Concepts and Controversies   Peter P. Toth and Kevin C. Maki
© 2008 John Wiley & Sons, Ltd

It is estimated that over 79 million American adults, or one in three, have one or more types of CVD [1]. Early, aggressive identification and management of patients at risk for CHD is essential to any effort aimed at reducing cardiovascular morbidity and mortality. The association between increased LDL-C and the development of CHD is widely acknowledged. Lowering LDL-C reduces the risk of coronary events, with greater LDL-C reduction leading to greater reduction in risk for events [2, 3]. This chapter reviews the management of LDL-C in both the primary and secondary prevention settings.

5.1 RELATIONSHIP BETWEEN LDL-C AND RISK FOR CARDIOVASCULAR EVENTS

LDL is the major atherogenic lipoprotein and LDL-C has long been identified as a primary target of cholesterol lowering therapy for reducing risk for CHD [4]. Data from cohort studies show a clear relationship between LDL-C and risk for CHD, MI, peripheral arterial disease, carotid artery disease (CAD) and ischemic stroke, and sudden death. The Framingham Heart Study [5], the Multiple Risk Factor Intervention Trial (MRFIT) [6], and the Lipid Research Clinics Coronary Primary Prevention Trial (LRC-CPPT) trial all identified a direct relationship between LDL-C and the incidence of new-onset CHD [7]. The Framingham Study demonstrated that among 2489 men and 2856 women aged 30–74 followed for 12 years, a total of 383 men and 227 women developed CHD and risk was significantly associated with blood pressure, total cholesterol (TC), LDL-C, and high-density lipoprotein cholesterol (HDL-C) (all $P < 0.001$) [5]. The adjusted attributable risk of CHD events associated with elevated TC (≥ 200 mg dl^{-1}) was 27% in men and 34% in women [5]. In MRFIT, a large cohort of 356 222 men aged 35–57 years, a significant relationship was found between serum cholesterol and CHD that was continuous and graded based on cholesterol quintiles. Of all CHD deaths, 46% were attributable to serum cholesterol levels ≥ 180 mg dl^{-1} [6]. The heightened risk for CVD as TC or LDL-C increase is remarkably consistent throughout most regions of the world [8–10].

The LRC-CPPT was a primary prevention study of 3806 men and demonstrated the efficacy of cholesterol lowering with cholestyramine, a BAS, for reducing CHD events. Cholestyramine therapy was associated with a 13.4% reduction in LDL-C and a 19% reduction in CHD events [7, 11]. The Scandinavian Simvastatin Survival Study (4S) further defined the importance of reducing LDL-C for secondary prevention of cardiovascular events. In 4S, 4444 patients with CHD were randomized to therapy with either placebo or 20–40 mg of simvastatin daily. The group treated with simvastatin experienced a 35% reduction in LDL-C and a 30% reduction in overall mortality compared to placebo. This was the first trial with a lipid-altering agent to demonstrate a statistically significant reduction in total

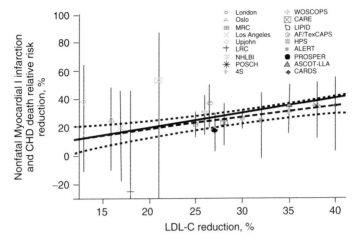

Figure 5.1 Meta-regression of prospective intervention trials evaluating the effect of low-density lipoprotein cholesterol (LDL-C) reduction on risk for cardiovascular events. Dotted lines represent 95% confidence intervals. Eighteen trials are included in this analysis. AF/TexCAPS, Air Force/Texas Coronary Atherosclerosis Prevention Study; ALERT, Assessment of LEscol in Renal Transplantation; ASCOT-LLA, Anglo-Scandinavian Cardiac Outcomes Trial–Lipid Lowering Arm; CARDS, Collaborative Atorvastatin Diabetes Study; CARE, Cholesterol and Recurrent Events study; HPS, Heart Protection Study; Los Angeles (Dayton *et al.* (1969) *Circulation*, **40** Suppl II:II1-63); LIPID, Long-Term Intervention with Pravastatin in Ischemic Disease; London Hospitals (*Lancet* (1965), **2**, 501-504); LRC, Lipid Research Clinics; MRC, Medical Research Council; NHLBI, National Heart, Lung, and Blood Institute; Oslo (*Acta Med Scand* (1966), **466**, 5-92); POSCH, Program on the Surgical Control of the Hyperlipidemias; PROSPER, PROspective Study of Pravastatin in the Elderly at Risk; 4S, Scandinavian Simvastatin Survival Study; Upjohn (Dorr *et al* (1978), *J Chron. Dis*, **31**, 5-14); WOSCOPS, West of Scotland Coronary Prevention Study. Data used with permission from Robinson, J.G. (2005) *Journal of the American College of Cardiology*, **46**, 1855–62, [13]. A full-color version of this figure appears in the color plate section of this book.

mortality. Based on the results of 4S, it was estimated that each 1% reduction in LDL-C reduces risk of CHD death and non-fatal MI by 1.7% [12]. A recent meta-regression of 10 placebo-controlled statin trials demonstrated that each 1% reduction in LDL-C lowered the relative risk of CHD death and non-fatal MI and stroke by 1% (Figure 5.1) [13]. The hazard for developing CHD or experiencing an acute CHD-related event approaches zero at an LDL-C level of approximately 40 mg dl^{-1} (Figure 5.2). Consequently, to a great degree, when it comes to LDL-C and risk reduction, it is generally accepted that "lower is better" [14].

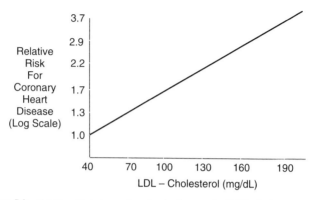

Figure 5.2 Relationship between low-density lipoprotein (LDL) cholesterol and risk for coronary heart disease. Reproduced with permission from Grundy, S.M. *et al.* (2004) *Journal of the American College of Cardiology*, **44**, 720–32, [2].

5.2 CLINICAL TRIAL SUPPORT FOR VERY AGGRESSIVE LDL-C REDUCTION FOR THOSE AT HIGHEST RISK

In 2004, updates to the NCEP ATP III guidelines added a category of "very high-risk" for patients with established CVD plus multiple major risk factors or severe, poorly controlled risk factors (e.g. diabetes or continued cigarette smoking), metabolic syndrome or acute coronary syndromes (Table 5.1) [2]. Persons with CHD or CHD risk equivalents have an LDL-C goal of <100 mg dl^{-1}, while very high-risk patients have an optional lower LDL-C goal of <70 mg dl^{-1} [2]. A systematic approach to LDL-C lowering in very high-risk patients is shown in Table 5.2.

Lowering LDL-C levels to levels substantially less than 100 mg dl^{-1} has shown incremental benefit in several clinical trials. The treating to new targets (TNT) trial included 10 001 patients with CHD and demonstrated that intensive statin therapy with atorvastatin 80 mg day^{-1} lowered the mean LDL-C level to 77 mg dl^{-1} compared with standard therapy of atorvastatin 10 mg day^{-1}, which lowered the mean LDL-C level to 101 mg dl^{-1} [18]. The lower LDL-C level with intensive statin therapy was associated with a 22% reduction in the relative risk of the primary composite endpoint, which included CHD death, non-fatal MI, resuscitated cardiac arrest, or fatal or non-fatal stroke (Table 5.3) [18]. Similarly, the Pravastatin or Atorvastatin Evaluation and Infection Therapy-Thrombolysis in Myocardial Infarction 22 (PROVE-IT) trial, which followed 4162 patients who had experienced recent acute coronary syndrome resulting in hospitalization, showed a decrease in the median LDL-C level to 62 mg dl^{-1} with

Table 5.1   Who is the high-risk patient?

CHD	• History of MI
	• Unstable angina
	• Stable angina
	• Angioplasty or bypass surgery
	• Clinically significant myocardial ischemia
CHD risk equivalents	• Peripheral arterial disease
	• Abdominal aortic aneurysm
	• Carotid artery disease (e.g. TIA, stroke, >50% obstruction of a carotid artery)
	• Diabetes mellitus
	• 2+ risk factors with >20% 10-yr risk for CHD
Very high-risk	Established CVD +
	• Multiple major risk factors (especially diabetes)
	• Severe and poorly controlled risk factors (especially continued cigarette smoking)
	• Multiple risk factors of the metabolic syndrome (especially TG $\geq$200 mg dl^{-1} + non-HDL-C $\geq$130 mg dl^{-1} with HDL-C <40 mg dl^{-1})
	• Acute coronary syndromes (unstable angina or acute MI)

CHD, coronary heart disease; CVD, cardiovascular disease; HDL-C, high-density lipoprotein cholesterol; MI, myocardial infarction; TG, triglycerides; TIA, transient ischemic attack. Adapted from data in Grundy, S.M. *et al.* (2004) *Circulation*, **110**, 227–39, [2], with additional data from Sarnak, M.J. *et al.* (2003) *Circulation*, **108**, 2154–69, [15].

Reproduced with permission from Toth, P.P. (2007) *Family Practice Recertification*, **29**, 24–37, [16].

intensive therapy (80 mg of atorvastatin daily) compared with 95 mg dl^{-1} in the moderate lipid-lowering therapy (40 mg of pravastatin daily) [19]. In PROVE-IT, the primary composite endpoint of all-cause mortality and cardiovascular events was reduced an additional 16% and the composite of all-cause mortality, non-fatal MI, and need for revascularization was reduced by an additional 25% in the group treated with high-dose atorvastatin relative to the pravastatin group.

The Heart Protection Study (HPS) examined the impact of simvastatin therapy (40 mg daily) in 20 536 high-risk persons with CHD, other occlusive

Table 5.2   How to treat very-high-risk patients to their LDL-C goal of <70 mg dl^{-1}.

- Consider intensive therapy for all patients admitted to the hospital with ACS
  - Measure LDL-C within 24 h of admission to determine drug choice and regimen
- Initiate statin therapy regardless of baseline LDL-C to obtain at least a 30–40% reduction in LDL-C
  - In patients with high baseline LDL-C
    - Use (or switch to) a powerful statin (e.g. atorvastatin, rosuvastatin)
    - If monotherapy is unsuccessful, try combination therapy with statin + ezetimibe or statin + niacin
  - In patients with LDL-C <100 mg dl^{-1} after standard-dose statin therapy
    - Use low dose of a more powerful statin or up-titrate standard regimen
- When triglycerides are elevated (≥200 mg dl^{-1}), use statin therapy to achieve a non–HDL-C level of 30 mg dl^{-1} above the LDL-C goal
  - When HDL-C is low and/or triglycerides are elevated, consider combination therapy with statin + niacin or statin + fenofibrate

---

Reproduced with permission from Toth, P.P. (2007) *Resident and Staff Physician*, **53**, s1–s7, [17].

arterial disease, or diabetes mellitus. Significant reductions in CHD event rates were seen in all subgroups, including those without diagnosed CHD but who had cerebrovascular disease, peripheral artery disease, or diabetes mellitus; men and women; those over or under age 70 years; and most notably, even in those who presented with a baseline LDL-C below 116 mg dl^{-1}. Among patients whose baseline LDL-C was already <100 mg dl^{-1}, there was an additional reduction of 20–30% in CHD risk with a 30% reduction in LDL-C [23]. The impact of greater LDL-C reduction on CHD-related event risk reduction was also confirmed in a recent meta-analysis of 14 randomized statin trials with 90 056 patients. This analysis showed a 12% reduction in all-cause mortality per 38.7 mg dl^{-1} reduction (1 mmol l^{-1}) in LDL-C [3]. For every millimolar per liter decrease in LDL-C, approximately 20% reductions were observed in the five-year incidence of MI or coronary death, need for coronary revascularization, and fatal or nonfatal stroke [3].

Table 5.3   The efficacy of statins in reducing CHD risk.

Primary prevention studies

Study	Drug	Design	Outcomes
AFCAPS/TexCAPS (1)	Lovastain, 20–40 mg d^{-1} vs placebo	6605 men and women	40% reduction in fatal and non-fatal MI; 37% reduction in first ACS; 33% reduction in coronary revascularizations; and unstable angina reduced by 32%
ASCOT (2)	Atorvastatin 10 mg d^{-1} vs placebo	10 305 hypertensive men ($n = 8463$) and women ($n = 1942$) with treated high BP and no previous CAD	36% reduction in total CHD/ non-fatal MI; 27% reduction in fatal and non-fatal stroke; total coronary event reduced by 29%; fatal and non-fatal stroke reduced by 27%
CARDS (3)	Atorvastatin 10 mg d^{-1} vs placebo	2838 patients with type 2 diabetes mellitus and 1 CHD risk factor(s)	37% reduction of major cardiovascular events; 27% of total mortality; 13.4% reduction of acute CVD events; 36% reduction of acute coronary events; 48% reduction of stroke
Heart Protection Study (4)	Simvastatin 40 mg d^{-1} vs placebo	20 536 high-risk (previous CHD, other vascular disease, hypertension among men aged > 65 yr, or diabetes)	25% reduction in all-cause and coronary death rates and in strokes; need for revacularisation reduced by 24%; fatal and non-fatal stroke reduced by 25%; non-fatal MI reduced by 38%; coronary mortality reduced by 18%; all cause mortality reduced by 13%; cardiovascular event rate reduced by 24%

(continued overleaf)

Table 5.3 *(continued)*

Primary prevention studies

Study	Drug	Design	Outcomes
PROSPER (5)	Pravastatin 40 mg d^{-1} vs pacebo	5804 men ($n = 2804$) and women ($n = 3000$) aged 70–82 yr	15% reduction in combined endpoint (fatal/non-fatal MI or stroke); 19% reduction in total/non-fatal CHD; no effect on stroke (but 25% reduction in TIA)
WOSCOPS (6)	Pravachol 40 mg d^{-1} vs placebo	6595 men	CHD death of non-fatal MI reduced by 31%; CVD death reduced by 32%; total mortality 22% reduction

Secondary prevention studies

Study	Drug	Design	Outcomes
4S (7)	Simvastatin 20 mg d^{-1} vs placebo	4444 pateints with angina pectoris or history of MI	Coronary mortality reduced by 42%; myocardial revascularization reduction of 37%; all cause mortality reduced by 30%; non-fatal major coronary event reduced by 34%; fatal and non-fatal stroke reduced by 30%

Table 5.3

Secondary prevention studies

Study	Drug	Design	Outcomes
AVERT (8)	Atorvastatin 80 mg d^{-1} vs angioplasty + usual care	341 patients with stable CAD	36% reduction in ischemic event; delayed time to first ischemic event reduced by 36%
CARE (9)	Pravastatin 40 mg d^{-1} vs placebo	3583 men and 576 women with history of MI	Death from CHD or non-fatal MI reduced by 24%; death from CHD reduced by 20%; non-fatal MI reduced by 23%; fatal MI reduced by 37%; CABG or PTCA reduced by 27%
LIPID (10)	Pravachol 40 mg d^{-1} vs placebo	9014 patients	Coronary mortality reduced by 24%; stroke reduced by 19%; fatal CHD or non-fatal MI reduced by 24%; fatal or non-fatal MI reduced by 29%
LIPS (11)	Fluvastatin 40 mg d^{-1} vs placebo	1667 men and women aged 18–80 yr postangioplasty for CAD	22% lower rate of major coronary events (e.g. cardiac deaths, non-fatal MI, or reintervention procedure)
MIRCAL (12)	Atorvastatin 80 mg d^{-1} vs placebo	3086 patients with ACS	Reduction in composite endpoint by 16%; ischemia reduced by 26%; stroke reduced by 50%
PROVE IT (13)	Atorvastatin 80 mg d^{-1} vs pravastatin 40 mg d^{-1}	4162 patients with ACS	16% reduction of composite endpoint; 14% reduction in CHD death, MI, or revascularization; revascularizations reduced by 14%; unstable angina reduced by 29%

(continued overleaf)

Table 5.3 (continued)

Secondary prevention studies

Study	Drug	Design	Outcomes
REVERSAL (14)	Atorvastatin 80 mg d^{-1} vs pravastatin 40 mg d^{-1}	654 patients with CAD	Atheroma: atorvastatin −0.4%, pravastatin 2.7%, difference of −3.1%, $p = 0.02$
TNT (15)	Atorvastatin 10 mg d^{-1} vs 80 mg d^{-1}	10 003 patients with CHD and LDL cholesterol 130–250 mg dL^{-1}	22% reduction in composite endpoint; MI reduced by 22%; stroke reduced by 25%

ACS, acute coronary syndrome; CABG, coronary artery bypass grafting; CAD, coronary artery disease; CHD, coronary heart disease; LDL, low-density lipoprotein; MI, myocardial infarction, PTCA, percutaneous translumenal coronay angioplasty.

Adapted from data in: Whitney, E. (1999) Current Atherosclerosis Reports, **1**, 38-43, [20].

Sever, P.S. et al. (2003) Lancet, **361**, 1149–58, [21].

Colhoun, H.M. et al. (2004) Lancet, **364**, 685–96, [22].

Heart Protection Study Collaborative Group. (2002) Lancet, **360**, 7–22, [23].

Shepherd, J. et al. (2002) Lancet, **360**, 1623–30, [24].

Shepherd, J., Cobbe, S.M., Ford, I. et al. (1995) The New England Journal of Medicine, **333**, 1301–07, [25].

Scandinavian Simvastatin Survival Study Group. (1994) Lancet, **344**, 1383–89, [26].

Pitt, B. et al. (1999) The New England Journal of Medicine, **341**, 70–76, [27].

Sacks, F.M. et al. (1996) The New England Journal of Medicine, **335**, 1001–9, [28].

The LIPID Study Group. (1995) The American Journal of Cardiology, **76**, 474–79, [29].

Serruys, P.W. et al. (2002) The Journal of the American Medical Association, **287**, 3215–22, [30].

Schwartz, G.G. et al. (2001) The Journal of the American Medical Association, **285**, 1711–18, [31].

Cannon, C.P. et al. (2004) The New England Journal of Medicine, **350**, 1495–504, [19].

Nissen, S. (2004) The Journal of the American Medical Association, **292**, 1–3, [32].

LaRosa, J.C. et al. (2005) The New England Journal of Medicine, **352**, 1425–35, [18].

Reproduced with permission from Toth, P.P. and Davidson, M.H. (2005) Expert Opinion on Pharmacotherapy, **6**, 131–139, [33].

5.3 GENETIC DISORDERS ASSOCIATED WITH ELEVATED LDL-C

An additional consideration in the assessment of patients with elevated LDL-C is that several genetic disorders cause elevated LDL-C, including FH, FCH, familial defective Apo B, and autosomal dominant hypercholesterolemia. FCH, an autosomal dominant disorder, is the most common genetic cause of elevated LDL-C [34]. In FCH, Apo B is overproduced, resulting in an abundance of very-low-density lipoprotein (VLDL) particles along with delayed clearance of postprandial triglycerides (TG) and an increased flux of free fatty acids [35]. The increase in VLDL particles leads to increased exchange of TG for cholesterol ester in high-density lipoprotein (HDL) or low-density lipoprotein (LDL) mediated by cholesterol ester transfer protein. The enrichment of these particles with TG renders them a better target for lipolysis by hepatic lipase, resulting in smaller HDL particles and smaller, denser LDL. As the HDL particles get progressively smaller, they became unstable and are ultimately catabolized. This gives rise to the so-called atherogenic lipid triad, of high TG, low HDL-C, and increased numbers of small, dense LDL particles (see Chapter 6 for more details on this phenotype).

5.4 ATHEROGENIC IMPACT OF LDL-C

LDL is considered to be the predominant atherogenic lipoprotein and high LDL concentrations initiate atherogenesis [36, 37]. The mechanisms through which LDL-C is atherogenic are complex. It is thought that circulating LDL particles filter into the arterial wall where they are trapped by intercellular matrix proteins and then undergo enzymatic oxidation and glycation. Modified LDL particles activate macrophages resident within the subendothelial space. Activated macrophages then express scavenging receptors such as CD36 and scavenging receptor A, which then bind and internalize LDL. As more and more lipid is taken up, the macrophage is converted into a foam cell. As foam cells coalesce, they help to form fatty streaks and atheromatous plaques (see Chapter 2 for additional detail on the atherogenic process).

LDL particles consist of several distinct subclasses that differ in size, density, and lipid content [38]. A predominance of smaller LDL particles, or phenotype B, is also associated with lower HDL and the cluster of abnormalities that characterize the metabolic syndrome, including insulin resistance, and increased risk of CVD [39]. Irrespective of LDL size, all LDL particles have the potential to be atherogenic within the arterial wall. Consistent with the latter statement, LDL particle number as measured by nuclear magnetic resonance spectroscopy, has a significant and continuous relationship with risk for acute cardiovascular events in both men and women [40–43].

Atherogenic dyslipidemia results in increased atherosclerotic plaque formation due to an imbalance between an increased number of small, dense LDL particles, which promote the deposition of cholesterol in the arterial wall, and the impaired removal of cholesterol secondary to low HDL. Cholesterol is also delivered into the arterial wall by other atherogenic lipoproteins, including VLDL, intermediate-density lipoprotein (IDL), and lipoprotein(a) [44].

Some patients can have genetic deficiencies of the LDL receptor (heterozygous and homozygous FH) leading to impaired clearance of atherogenic lipoproteins [45]. Many mutations leading to the phenotype of FH have been described [46]. Clinical features of FH, particularly among homozygotes, include corneal arcus, plantar and periosteal xanthomas, and increased prevalence of premature multivessel CAD [47]. Patients homozygous for FH frequently require LDL apheresis in order to significantly reduce serum LDL-C levels [48].

5.5   MANAGEMENT OF ELEVATED LDL-C

The management of elevated LDL-C is focused on instituting TLC, followed by pharmacologic therapy if necessary to achieve LDL-C treatment targets. TLC is described in detail in Chapter 4.

Statin therapy is most commonly used to reduce elevated LDL-C and to improve all components of the lipid profile. Statins have important lipid effects beyond LDL-C reduction that may also contribute to CVD risk reduction, including decreasing hepatic VLDL secretion (which results in lower serum TG levels) and raising HDL-C [49]. Other widely used lipid-altering drugs used in the management of elevated LDL-C include cholesterol absorption inhibitors (ezetimibe) and bile acid resins.

STATINS

The statins are the most widely used pharmacologic agents for the treatment of dyslipidemia. The statins are reversible, competitive inhibitors of 3-hydroxy-3-methlyglutarl coenzyme A (HMG-CoA) reductase, the rate-limiting enzyme for hepatic cholesterol biosynthesis.

In addition to reducing cholesterol biosynthesis, the statins enhance the clearance of atherogenic Apo B-100-containing lipoproteins (VLDL, VLDL remnants, and LDL) by upregulating the expression of the LDL receptor on the surface of hepatocytes. The statins stimulate Apo A-I expression and hepatic HDL secretion secondary to weak peroxisomal proliferator-activated receptor $-\alpha$ (PPAR $-\alpha$) agonism [50]. Statins also appear to exert benefits (pleiotropic effects) beyond decreasing circulating levels of atherogenic lipoproteins through anti-inflammatory effects and atheromatous plaque stabilization (Figure 5.3) [51]. Pleiotropic effects bring about a reduction in the production of a large number of atherogenic stimuli such as C-reactive protein, reactive oxygen species (superoxide anion, hydroxyl radical, peroxynitrite), tissue factor, interleukins, endothelial cell adhesion molecules, monocyte chemoattract protein-1, angiotensin-II receptor, and endothelin-1, as well as a decrease in platelet reactivity and smooth-cell proliferation, and a reversal of endothelial dysfunction, among others. As a result, the statins have been associated with modulating numerous mechanisms that reduce atherogenesis [52] and even stimulate its regression [53].

The various statins differ in their pharmacokinetic properties and potency. Lovastatin, simvastatin, and atorvastatin are metabolized via the cytochrome P450 (CYP) 3A4 pathway and as a result have the potential for drug interactions with agents that inhibit the CYP34A pathway. Fluvastatin is metabolized by the 2C9 pathway, and pravastatin and rosuvastatin are not significantly metabolized by the CYP pathway. The LDL-C reducing effect of the statins ranges from 45 to 63% for rosuvastatin (Crestor, 5–40 mg day^{-1}), 26 to 60% for atorvastatin (Lipitor, 10–80 mg day^{-1}), 26 to 47% for simvastatin (Zocor, 10–80 mg day^{-1}), 21 to 42% for lovastatin (Mevacor, 10–80 mg day^{-1}), 22 to 36% for fluvastatin (Lescol, 10–80 mg day^{-1}), and 22 to 34% for pravastatin (Pravachol, 10–80 mg day^{-1}).

A number of randomized large-scale, placebo-controlled trials in both the primary and secondary prevention settings have demonstrated the efficacy of statins in reducing CHD risk (see Table 5.3 for summary). The Air Force/Texas Coronary Atherosclerosis Prevention Study AFCAPS/TexCAPS [55] evaluated the use of lovastatin (20–40 mg day^{-1}) for the prevention of first acute major coronary event in 5608 men and 997 women without clinically evident atherosclerotic CHD and with average levels of TC and LDL-C, but below-average HDL-C. After a median follow-up of five years, lovastatin lowered LDL-C by an average of 25% to 115 mg dl^{-1} and significantly reduced the incidence of first acute coronary events (fatal or non-fatal MI ($P = 0.002$), unstable angina ($P = 0.02$), need for coronary revascularization procedures ($P = 0.001$), coronary events ($P = 0.006$), and cardiovascular events ($P = 0.003$) [55]. Another primary prevention trial, the Anglo-Scandinavian Cardiac Outcomes Trial-Lipid Lowering Arm (ASCOT-LLA) [21], examined the use of atorvastatin 10 mg day^{-1} in hypertensive patients with three or more other risk factors (e.g. family history of premature CAD, microalbuminuria, low HDL-C, left ventricular hypertrophy, etc.) with TC levels of 250 mg dl^{-1} or less. After a median follow-up of 3.3 years, atorvastatin lowered total serum cholesterol by 50 mg dl^{-1} at 12 months and by 43 mg dl^{-1} after

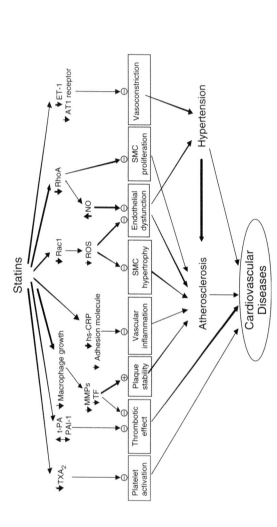

Figure 5.3 Pleiotropic effects of statins. In addition to their effects on cholesterol biosynthesis and capacity to beneficially impact serum concentrations of lipoproteins, the statins exert a variety of pleiotropic effects along blood vessel wall. It is believed that the statins reduce platelet aggregability, reverse endothelial dysfunction, promote vasodilatation, reduce inflammatory tone, and stabilize atheromatous plaque. AT1, angiotensin-II type 1 receptor; ET-1, endothelin type 1 receptor; hs-CRP, high-sensitivity C-reactive protein; MMP, matrix metalloproteinase; NO, nitric oxide; PAI-1, plasminogen activator inhibitor; Rac1, Ras-related C3 botulinum toxin substrate 1; RhoA, Ras homolog gene family, member A; ROS, reactive oxygen species; TF, tissue factor; t-PA, tissue plasminogen activator; TXA$_2$, thromboxane A$_2$. Reproduced with permission from Takemoto, M. and Liao, J.K. (2001) *Arteriosclerosis, Thrombosis, and Vascular Biology*, **21**, 1712–19, [54].

3 years of follow-up [21]. There were significant reductions in the primary composite endpoint (non-fatal MI and fatal CHD events; 36%, $P = 0.0005$), MI (45%, $P = 0.0002$), and fatal and nonfatal stroke (27%, $P = 0.024$). ASCOT-LLA was stopped nearly 2 years early by the study's Data Safety Monitoring Board because after only 3.3 years, the benefit of statin therapy was so strong they believed it would have been unethical to continue to withhold statin therapy from the placebo group.

In the Collaborative Atorvastatin Diabetes Study (CARDS) [22], 2838 patients with type 2 diabetes mellitus but no history of CHD were randomized to therapy with either atorvastatin 10 mg daily or placebo. In these patients, atorvastatin therapy was associated with significant reductions in the primary composite endpoint of acute CHD events (36%, $P = 0.001$), MI (42%, $P = 0.007$), and fatal/non-fatal stroke (48%, $P = 0.007$) after a median follow-up of 3.9 years. CARDS was also stopped approximately two years earlier than planned because of the magnitude of benefit in the atorvastatin group compared with the placebo group. The West of Scotland Coronary Prevention Study (WOSCOPS) [25] evaluated the efficacy of pravastatin 40 mg day^{-1} in 6595 men with hypercholesterolemia and no history of previous MI. After an average of 4.9 years of follow-up, pravastatin lowered plasma TC by 20% and LDL-C by 26%, and significantly reduced risk of non-fatal MI (31%, $P < 0.001$), death from CHD (28%, $P = 0.13$), and death from all cardiovascular causes (32%, $P = 0.0033$) [25].

Various secondary prevention clinical trials have demonstrated the benefit of statin therapy including 4S [12], Cholesterol and Recurrent Events (CARE) [28]. Long-term Intervention with Pravastatin in Ischaemic Disease (LIPID) [56], HPS [23], A to Z trial [57], TNT [58], Incremental Decrease in End Points Through Aggressive Lipid Lowering (IDEAL) [59], and the Pravastatin in Elderly Individuals at Risk of Vascular Disease (PROSPER) [24]. These trials have affirmed the central concept that the greatest absolute benefit from LDL-C reduction accrues to those with the highest absolute risk, emphasizing the importance of aggressive lipid management in secondary prevention (see Chapter 1, Figure 1.1).

EZETIMIBE

Ezetimibe (Zetia) is the first member of a class of lipid-lowering drugs known as *cholesterol absorption inhibitors* [60]. Ezetimibe localizes to the brush border of jejunal enterocytes and inhibits the uptake of biliary and dietary sources of cholesterol (Figure 5.4). Ezetimibe specifically binds to the Nieman Pick C1 like-1 sterol transporter [61]. Ezetimibe does not affect the absorption of TG, fatty acids, bile acids, or fat-soluble vitamins, including vitamins A, D, E, and α and β-carotenes [62, 63]. After oral administration, ezetimibe is rapidly glucuronidated in the intestines and subsequently undergoes enterohepatic recirculation, resulting in a repeated

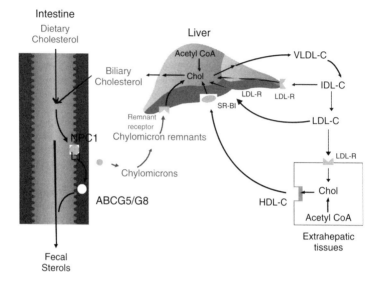

Figure 5.4 Cholesterol absorption, hepatic biosynthesis, and systemic distribution. Cholesterol enters the gastrointestinal tract from both dietary and biliary sources. Cholesterol is solubilized into micelles with bile salts and lipids. Micelles interact with enterocytes along the brush border of the jejunum. The sterol transporter Nieman Pick C1-like 1 protein (NPC1) binds and transports cholesterol and phytosterols into the enterocyte's interior. This transporter is inhibited by the drug ezetimibe. Phtyosterols are typically transported back into the intestinal lumen via the ABCG5/G8 heterodimer. ABCG5/G8 can also translocate excess cholesterol out of the enterocyte. Absorbed sterols are esterified and combined with apoprotein B48 and other lipids to form chylomicrons. Chylomicrons are secreted into the enterolymph and gain access into the central circulation via the thoracic duct. Chylomicrons deliver cholesterol and triglycerides to the liver. Cholesterol and triglycerides can then be packaged into VLDL and secreted by the liver. The triglycerides in VLDL are hydrolyzed by lipoprotein lipase progressively yielding IDL and then LDL. The LDL particles can either be taken up into arterial walls or can be taken up by the liver by LDL receptors. A full-color version of this figure appears in the color plate section of this book.

delivery of the drug to its site of action, with minimal systemic exposure [64]. The timing of dosing does not affect its activity [65] and food does not affect its bioavailability [66].

Ezetimibe has been demonstrated to reduce LDL-C on average by 18–20% (the equivalent of three statin titration steps) and has established efficacy as monotherapy in reducing LDL-C in patients with hypercholesterolemia [67, 68], as well as in combination therapy with statins [69–72]. Coadministration of ezetimibe with atorvastatin and simvastatin 10, 20, 40, or 80 mg and with lovastatin and pravastatin 10, 30, or 40 mg resulted in more effective LDL-C lowering than with a statin alone at each statin dose level. Notably, coadministration of ezetimibe 10 mg daily with the lowest statin dose was as effective as statin monotherapy at the highest dose and the efficacy of coadministration therapy was not influenced by age, race, gender, or level of CHD risk [49].

A fixed-dose combination of ezetimibe with increasing doses of simvastatin is available (Vytorin; 10/10; 10/20; 10/40; 10/80 mg daily) [33]. The addition of ezetimibe to statin therapy can reduce the likelihood of having to titrate the statin. The coadministration of ezetimibe to statin therapy is well tolerated and generally has an adverse event profile similar to statin monotherapy [69–72]. To date, no cases of hepatitis, jaundice, or other clinical signs of liver dysfunction have been reported with ezetimibe–statin combination therapy. Ezetimibe is also indicated for the treatment of the rare disorder β-sitosterolemia. In β-sitosterolemia, patients are afflicted with mutations in the membrane casette transport protein heterodimer ABCG5/G8, a translocase responsible for externalizing excess intracellular cholesterol and plant sterols or phytosterols (e.g. sitosterol, campesterol) from the cytosol of enterocytes [73]. In patients with β-sitosterolemia, high levels of phytosterols are atherogenic and can induce premature CAD, especially in homozygotes. Ezetimibe has not yet been shown to reduce risk for cardiovascular events, though multiple trials are ongoing to further evaluate this issue.

BILE ACID SEQUESTRANTS

BASs or bile acid binding resins are orally administered anion exchange resins that bind bile acids in the gastrointestinal (GI) tract and prevent their reabsorption into the enterohepatic circulation via the ileal bile acid transport protein [74]. BASs reduce LDL-C by increasing the catabolism of cholesterol, secondary to the upregulation of 7-α-hydroxylase, a rate-limiting enzyme for the conversion of cholesterol into bile acids; and by increasing the expression of LDL receptors on the hepatocyte surface, thereby enhancing the clearance of Apo B-100-containing lipoproteins from plasma. BASs are used as monotherapy or, more often, as part of combination therapy with a statin for the management of dyslipidemia. Of the BASs, cholestyramine (Questran) and colestipol (Colestid) have proven to be effective and safe non-systemic approaches to LDL-C reduction; however, tolerability and compliance issues related to palatability and GI side effects have limited their use. Colesevelam hydrochloride (WelChol) is effective in reducing LDL-C (12–20%) in patients with mild to moderate hypercholesterolemia. The lipid-lowering effects of BASs are attributed to the increasing hepatic conversion of intracellular cholesterol to bile acids, altered hepatic intracellular cholesterol distribution, and enhanced clearance of serum LDL-C due to upregulation in the expression of hepatic LDL receptors [75].

The clinical benefit of BASs was demonstrated in the Lipid Research Clinics Coronary Primary Prevention Trial [7, 11], which showed that cholestyramine dosed at 24 g day^{-1} significantly reduced LDL-C in 3806 middle-aged men with primary hypercholesterolemia (type II hyperlipoproteinemia). Men in the cholestyramine treated group showed an 8.5% greater reduction in TC and 12.6% greater reduction in LDL-C compared with placebo. They also experienced a 19% reduction in risk of CHD death and/or non-fatal MI [7, 11]. Colesevelam HCl was demonstrated to be effective as monotherapy and in statin combination therapy with lovastatin [76], simvastatin [77], and atorvastatin [78]. BAS therapy increases HMG-CoA reductase activity in the liver, leading to increased hepatic biosynthesis of cholesterol. Thus, the combination of a BAS with statin therapy is an attractive approach.

BASs have been associated with high rates of discontinuation (40–60%) due to poor palatability of the drug and to the occurrence of GI adverse effects, especially constipation [79]. Constipation is the most common adverse effect for BASs, occurring in 10% of patients taking colestipol and in up to 28% of patients taking cholestyramine [80]. Colesevelam HCl tends not to constipate patients as it forms a soft gel while in transit through the GI tract. The BASs can reduce the absorption of fat-soluble vitamins, warfarin, phenobarbital, thiazide diuretics, digitalis, β-blockers, thyroxine, statins, fibrates, and ezetimibe. These agents should be administered 1 hour before or 4 hours after ingestion of a BASs. Agents in the BAS class can also induce paradoxical elevations in serum TG for reasons that are poorly understood.

NIACIN AND FIBRATES

Niacin and fibrates are most commonly used for the treatment of hypertriglyceridemia and/or low HDL-C (often in combination with another agent) and are covered in more detail in Chapters 6 and 7. However, both drugs have moderate capacity to lower LDL-C (5–20%), particularly in mixed dyslipidemias in which the patient has disturbances in LDL-C combined with hypertriglyceridemia and/or depressed HDL-C. Clinicians should be aware that the effects of fibrates (fenofibrate and gemfibrozil) on LDL-C are highly dependent on the pretreatment TG concentration. When TG are ≥350 mg dl^{-1}, LDL-C may rise with fibrate therapy, whereas LDL-C is more likely to be reduced when the starting TG level is lower. In part, this reflects impaired conversion of VLDL to LDL particles in patients with marked hypertriglyceridemia, which is partially normalized when the TG level is lowered during fibrate therapy. Both fibrates and niacin have been found to reduce CHD event risk and progression of coronary atherosclerosis in clinical trials [4].

POTENTIAL TOXICITIES OF LIPID-LOWERING MEDICATIONS

While the efficacy of statin therapy in the management of CHD is well established, statin use can be associated with an elevation in liver transaminase levels. The responsible mechanisms for this phenomenon are not well established. Elevations in the liver enzymes alanine aminotransferase (ALT) or aspartate aminotransferase (AST) can occur with statin therapy but are often transient and resolve spontaneously [81]. Recommendations of the National Lipid Association Statin Safety Assessment Task Force reinforce the initial and continued monitoring of liver transaminase levels for elevation to ensure safety in the use of statin therapy [81]. Liver function tests (LFTs) should be measured at baseline and then 6–12 weeks after initiating statin therapy and 6–12 weeks after dose titrations. Patients typically find reassurance if their provider then monitors LFTs twice yearly once a stable dose has been achieved. Hepatotoxicity is defined as an elevation in liver transaminase levels ≥three times the upper limit of normal on two occasions measured at least one month apart. If this threshold is reached, statin therapy should be discontinued until LFTs normalize. At that point, a different statin can be initiated or a rechallenge with the same statin at a lower dose can also be considered.

Myopathy, defined as a creatine kinase elevation 10 times the upper limit of normal with associated muscle pain or weakness, can also occur with statin therapy [82]. The most serious side effect of statin therapy is rhabdomyolysis in which skeletal muscle breakdown, myoglobinuria, and renal failure occur. This constitutes a medical emergency. The risk is well below 1%; however, patients should be instructed on the signs and symptoms of rhabdomyolysis, including increasing muscle pain, weakness, and brownish-red discoloration of urine. Myalgia is likely the most common adverse side-effect associated with statin therapy. Complaints of myalgia should be investigated with a careful history and physical examination. Measuring a serum creatine kinase level is usually not necessary. However, if the patient is complaining of escalating muscle pain (which can be either uni- or bilateral in distribution) with weakness, then consideration should be given to the measurement of serum creatine kinase levels.

There are no prospective, placebo-controlled clinical trials evaluating the capacity of exogenous coenzyme Q10 to reduce or prevent myalgias. However, if a patient is experiencing recurrent myalgias on multiple statins, consideration can be given to CoQ10 supplementation at 100–200 mg daily [83]. In some cases this has been found to ameliorate muscle pain. Other potential causes of the myopathy include drug interaction (e.g. another drug is inhibiting the metabolism and clearance of the statin), thyroid dysfunction, renal insufficiency, and electrolyte disturbances, all of which should also be carefully ruled out. The mechanisms modulating statin-induced myopathy are heterogeneous and identifying specific etiologies is still investigational [84–86]. It is well documented that occasionally statin therapy will unmask established, underlying myopathy in some patients.

5.6 SUMMARY

The high prevalence of CVD and all forms of atherosclerotic disease mandates a targeted, systematic approach to reducing risk. LDL-C reduction is a central component of risk reduction strategies [16, 17]. The management of elevated LDL-C with lifestyle modifications and pharmacologic therapy has proven to be efficacious and associated with reductions in risk for a broad variety of cardiovascular endpoints, including MI, stroke, angina pectoris, and death. NCEP ATP III provides evidence-based guidance on the appropriate clinical approach to managing dyslipidemia based on quantitative risk assessment.

Evidence from a number of clinical trials, both primary and secondary prevention based, support the beneficial effects of statins for reducing CHD and cardiovascular event risk, and statins are recognized as a first-line treatment for dyslipidemia. Other pharmacologic agents for targeting LDL-C reduction include the cholesterol absorption inhibitor ezetimibe and BASs, including colesevelam HCl. Statin therapy used in combination with these agents has demonstrated efficacy, particularly in patients who have not achieved NCEP ATP III goals with maximal statin therapy or a maximally tolerated dose.

CONTROVERSY

HOW LOW SHOULD WE GO?

Are There Risks Associated with a Very Low Serum Level of LDL-C?

Recent clinical trials strongly support the conclusion that, when it comes to serum levels of LDL-C, lower is better. More aggressive reductions in LDL-C have been shown to provide statistically greater reductions in cardiovascular morbidity and mortality. This conclusion is supported by such studies as PROVE-IT TIMI 22, TNT, IDEAL, and A to Z [1–4]. In PROVE-IT and TNT, high-dose statin therapy with atorvastatin 80 mg daily reduced serum LDL-C to mean levels of 62 mg dl^{-1} and 75 mg dl^{-1}, respectively. These levels are substantially lower than that advocated by the NCEP ATP III for high risk patients. Both demonstrated significant reductions in their primary composite endpoints with greater LDL-C lowering without increasing adverse events. In IDEAL and A–Z, the primary composite endpoints did not achieve statistical significance. However, in IDEAL, multiple secondary endpoints, including non-fatal myocardial infarction, peripheral arterial disease, and need for revascularization via coronary angionplasty or bypass grafting were significantly reduced when comparing atorvastatin 80 mg to moderate doses (20–40 mg) of simvastatin (mean attained LDL-C levels of 81 and 104 mg dl^{-1}, respectively). In the A–Z trial, during the final 20 months, high-dose simvastatin therapy (80 mg) reduced cardiovascular events 25% more than the comparator dose (20 mg) of this statin, despite the fact that the attained serum LDL-C in the two groups were not markedly different: 67 and 81 mg dl^{-1}, respectively. In aggregate, the results from the outcome trials mentioned above are consistent with those from REVERSAL [5] and ASTEROID [6], which used coronary intravascular ultrasonography to assess responses to statin therapy and attained LDL-C 78 and 61 mg dl^{-1}, respectively. These trials showed that more aggressive lipid therapy was associated with less plaque progression and even plaque regression in some subjects. High-dose statin therapy has been shown to have an acceptable benefit to risk ratio [7].

Historically, there has been some concern that if serum cholesterol was lowered too aggressively, this could adversely impact lipid and sterol metabolism. We appear to have a much better understanding of this now, though there is still much to be learned. An infant is typically born with a serum LDL-C of 30–40 mg dl^{-1}. During the neonatal period, this level of LDL-C certainly appears to suffice for metabolic needs and the requirements for normal neurologic and other patterns of development and growth.

Very little of the cholesterol in the central circulation crosses the blood-brain barrier. Virtually all of the cholesterol in the human brain is produced by the brain [8]. Importantly, there is no indication to date that lowering serum cholesterol is associated with premature neurologic degeneration. Reducing LDL-C is unlikely to adversely impact steroid hormone biosynthesis since HDL is the lipoprotein that delivers cholesterol to steroidogenic organs such as the placenta, ovaries, testes, and adrenal glands. The average total cholesterol of modern-day hunter-gatherer peoples is approximately 110 mg dl^{-1} [9]. This is substantially lower than the average total cholesterol of 210 mg dl^{-1} in American adults. Hunter-gatherers lived and adapted to their environment during the late Paleolithic period, which lasted hundreds of thousands of years. The agricultural revolution began $\sim$10 000 years ago, while the industrial revolution began in England only a bit more than 200 years ago. In this context, it is clear that humans spent most of their evolutionary history adapting to a hunter-gatherer lifestyle. We have simply not had enough time to develop and naturally select mutations in lipid and sterol metabolism that would make us more apt to physiologically cope with and survive the exposure to environmental changes wrought by the industrial/technologic age in which we now live. This is amply substantiated by the incidence of atherosclerotic disease in the western world. Cholesterol is among the most important toxins we are exposed to in our lifetime. It makes intuitive sense to try to minimize systemic exposure to such an important and ubiquitous toxin which we ingest and endogenously produce every day of our lives.

The relationship between serum LDL-C and absolute risk for CHD is curvilinear (or linear if expressed on a log scale) [10]. Risk reduction becomes progressively more attenuated as LDL-C is pushed to lower and lower levels. However, risk does continue to decrease. In a recent post hoc analysis of data from the PROVE-IT trial, as LDL-C decreased to <40 mg dl^{-1}, cardiovascular risk was less than that seen at 60–80 mg dl^{-1} with no increase in noncardiovascular adverse events [11]. The NCEP estimates that there is no excess risk for a CHD related event at a serum LDL-C of 40 mg dl^{-1} [12]. Is there other evidence to suggest this may be a safe level to attain? In patients with hypobetalipoproteinemia, it is not unusual to observe lifelong serum LDL-C levels of 25–50 mg dl^{-1}. This is associated with longevity. In patients with loss of function mutations in PCSK9, the LDL receptor is not cleared from the hepatocyte cell membrane in a normal manner. These patients experience lifelong upregulation of the LDL receptor with significant reductions in serum LDL-C and decreased risk for cardiovascular events compared to patients with normal PCSK9 function [13]. In a meta-analysis of 14 statin trials, the 'Cholesterol Treatment Trialists' Collaboration found no evidence for increased risk for cancer or hemorrhagic stroke [14]. Although concern about increased risk for hemorrhagic stroke dates back to the Multiple Risk Factor Intervention Trial [15], the more recent SPARCL study showed that, among patients on high-dose atorvastatin therapy, increased risk for hemorrhagic stroke was associated with inadequate blood pressure control and a prior history of hemorrhagic stroke, not LDL-C reduction [16, 17]. To date, there are no adequately documented risks or forms of toxicity when LDL-C is lowered into the 40–60 mg dl^{-1} range or less. In fact, patients with lifelong very low levels of LDL-C (25–40 mg dl^{-1}) have reduced vulnerability to the development of atherosclerotic disease.

So, how low do you go? We do not have adequate clinical trial data to answer this question in a scientifically rigorous manner. We do not know if there is a lower threshold below which little to no additional risk reduction can be obtained. There also does not appear to be undue risk for morbidity and mortality when LDL-C is chronically very low. However, a variety of epidemiologic and subgroup analyses from completed clinical trials paint a consistent picture: when it comes to LDL-C, lower is better if the goal is to reduce risk for atherosclerotic disease progression and decrease risk for cardiovascular morbidity and mortality. Patients who may be most appropriately targeted for *very low* LDL-C (i.e. 35–60 mg dl^{-1}) may include those who attain all of their national guideline stated goals for lipids, blood pressure, exercise, weight loss, glycemic control, and smoking cessation, yet still sustain a breakthrough cardiovascular event. Patients who have required revascularization, who have multivessel CAD, or who have had an ACS may also be good candidates for very aggressive LDL-C reduction. Until we have more clinical trial evidence, this appears to be a reasonable approach and one that would serve our patients' best interests, as long as they can tolerate their lipid-lowering regimens.

REFERENCES

[1] Cannon, C.P., Braunwald, E., McCabe, C.H. *et al*. (2004) Intensive versus moderate lipid lowering with statins after acute coronary syndromes. *The New England Journal of Medicine*, **350**, 1495–504.

[2] LaRosa, J.C., Grundy, S.M., Waters, D.D. *et al*. (2005) Intensive lipid lowering with atorvastatin in patients with stable coronary disease. *The New England Journal of Medicine*, **352**, 1425–35.

[3] Pedersen, T., Faergeman, O., Kastelein, J. *et al*. (2005) High-dose atorvastatin versus usual-dose simvastatin for secondary prevention after myocardial infarction: the IDEAL study: a randomized controlled trial. *The Journal of the American Medical Association*, **294**, 2437–45.

[4] de Lemos, J.A., Blazing, M.A., Wiviott, S.D. *et al*. (2004) Early intensive vs a delayed conservative simvastatin strategy in patients with acute coronary syndromes: phase Z of the A to Z trial. *The Journal of the American Medical Association*, **292**, 1307–16.
[5] Nissen, S.E., Tuzcu, E.M., Schoenhagen, P. *et al*. (2004) Effect of intensive compared with moderate lipid-lowering therapy on progression of coronary atherosclerosis: a randomized controlled trial. *The Journal of the American Medical Association*, **291**, 1071–80.
[6] Nissen, S.E., Nicholls, S.J., Sipahi, I. *et al*. (2006) Effect of very high-intensity statin therapy on regression of coronary atherosclerosis: the ASTEROID trial. *The Journal of the American Medical Association*, **295**, 1556–65.
[7] Davidson, M.H. and Robinson, J.G. (2007) Safety of aggressive lipid management. *Journal of the American College of Cardiology*, **49**, 1753–62.
[8] Bjorkhem, I. and Meaney, S. (2004) Brain cholesterol: long secret life behind a barrier. *Arteriosclerosis, Thrombosis, and Vascular Biology*, **24**, 806–15.
[9] O'Keefe, J.H. Jr, Cordain, L., Harris, W.H. *et al*. (2004) Optimal low-density lipoprotein is 50 to 70mg/dl: lower is better and physiologically normal. *Journal of the American College of Cardiology*, **43**, 2142–46.
[10] Stamler, J., Wentworth, D. and Neaton, J.D. (1986) Is relationship between serum cholesterol and risk of premature death from coronary heart disease continuous and graded? Findings in 356,222 primary screenees of the Multiple Risk Factor Intervention Trial (MRFIT). *The Journal of the American Medical Association*, **256**, 2823–28.
[11] Wiviott, S.D., Cannon, C.P., Morrow, D.A. *et al*. (2005) Can low-density lipoprotein be too low? The safety and efficacy of achieving very low low-density lipoprotein with intensive statin therapy: a PROVE IT-TIMI 22 substudy. *Journal of the American College of Cardiology*, **46**, 1411–16.
[12] Grundy, S.M., Cleeman, J.I., Merz, C.N., *et al*. (2004) Implications of recent clinical trials for the National Cholesterol Education Program Adult Treatment Panel III guidelines. *Circulation*, **110**, 227–39.
[13] Cohen, J.C., Boerwinkle, E., Mosley, T.H. Jr and Hobbs, H.H. (2006) Sequence variations in PCSK9, low LDL, and protection against coronary heart disease. *The New England Journal of Medicine*, **354**, 1264–72.
[14] Baigent, C., Keech, A., Kearney, P.M. *et al*. (2005) Efficacy and safety of cholesterol-lowering treatment: prospective meta-analysis of data from 90,056 participants in 14 randomised trials of statins. *Lancet*, **366**, 1267–78.
[15] Neaton, J.D., Blackburn, H., Jacobs, D. *et al*. (1992) Serum cholesterol level and mortality findings for men screened in the Multiple Risk Factor Intervention Trial. Multiple Risk Factor Intervention Trial Research Group. *Archives of Internal Medicine*, **152**, 1490–500.

[16] Amarenco, P., Bogousslavsky, J., Callahan, A., III *et al*. (2006) High-dose atorvastatin after stroke or transient ischemic attack. *The New England Journal of Medicine*, **355**, 549–59.

[17] Armani, A. and Toth, P.P. (2007) SPARCL: the glimmer of statins for stroke risk reduction. *Current Atherosclerosis Reports*, **9**, 347–51.

CONTROVERSY

RISKS AND BENEFITS OF HIGH-DOSE STATIN THERAPY VERSUS COMBINATION LIPID DRUG THERAPY

Lipoprotein metabolism is quite complex and many forms of dyslipidemia have been biochemically characterized. The NCEP ATP III goals for lipid lowering are well defined and based on quantitative risk stratification [1, 2]. It is widely acknowledged that reducing the atherogenic lipoprotein burden in serum (i.e. LDL-C and non-HDL-C) is critically important to any risk reduction strategy. Similarly, NCEP recommends that when serum concentrations of HDL-C are low, therapies be instituted that raise levels of this lipoprotein. Statins are among the most intensively investigated medications in the history of medicine. Their safety profile has been validated throughout the world in men and women, the young and the elderly, and in patients of many racial and ethnic groups. Statins are the drug of choice for LDL-C reduction. They also have variable capacity to lower serum TG and raise HDL-C in a drug and dose-dependent manner [3, 4]. However, even at maximal doses of statins, many patients will not be able to achieve their comprehensive NCEP lipoprotein targets. In these situations, it is of course reasonable to try to tailor combinations of drugs which may normalize multiple components of the lipid profile. Appropriate candidates for combination therapy include patients who: (i) cannot tolerate statin titration secondary to myalgias or serum transaminase elevations or refusal to take a higher dose; (ii) cannot achieve their lipoprotein targets on high-dose statin monotherapy; (iii) have insulin resistance states such as metabolic syndrome and diabetes mellitus; and (iv) have inborn errors of lipid metabolism, such as familial combined hyperlipidemia, familial hypercholesterolemia, familial hypoalphalipoproteinemia (severe low HDL-C), and severe hypertriglyceridemia secondary to mutations in lipoprotein lipase or apoproteins CII and CIII. In patients with baseline fasting TG >500 mg dl^{-1}, the use of combination therapy to normalize serum TG is almost always necessary. In patients with severe hypertriglyceridemia, the goal is to prevent pancreatitis and development/progression of non-alcoholic hepatic steatosis, not just cardiovascular events.

When considering combination therapy, it is important to assess whether or not specific approaches are efficacious and evidence-based. In addition, a crucial consideration is whether or not combination therapy has demonstrated safety in both the near and long-term. For the most part, the majority of the endpoint-driven, prospective, long-term clinical trials performed since the early 1990s have tested the efficacy of single agent therapy in both the primary and secondary prevention settings. High-dose statin therapy has demonstrated efficacy for reducing cardiovascular morbidity and mortality [5, 6] and safety [7]. The best studied combination therapy to date is the coadministration of a statin with niacin in patients with established CAD. In the HATS trial, the combination of a statin with niacin significantly reduced the primary composite endpoint and rates of coronary atherosclerotic disease progression [8]. In ARBITER 2, statin/niacin combination therapy reduced rates of progression of carotid atherosclerotic disease [9]. The capacity of niacin to augment the ability of statin therapy to beneficially impact the course of atherosclerotic disease is being tested in a larger cohort of patients in the AIM-HIGH trial. In the meantime, the addition of niacin to statin therapy improves all components of the lipid profile (decreases in LDL-C, TG, non-HDL-C, and Lp(a), and increases HDL-C). Niacin can dramatically augment the beneficial effects of a statin on serum lipid levels.

There are no endpoint trials currently completed that establish the efficacy of combining a statin with a fibrate, ezetimibe, omega-3 fish oils, or a bile acid binding resin. The ACCORD trial is underway and is comparing the capacity of simvastatin monotherapy with simvastatin/fenofibrate combination therapy to reduce risk for acute cardiovascular events in patients with diabetes mellitus. This trial will not likely conclude until 2010. It is generally agreed that the use of fenofibrate in combination with a statin is safer and entails a substantially lower risk for rhabdomyolysis than combination therapy with gemfibrozil [10, 11]. The IMPROVE-IT trial is comparing simvastatin monotherapy with simvastatin/ezetimibe combination therapy in patients with CAD. It will likely be completed in 2011. Although it is complicated by numerous methodological difficulties, the ENHANCE trial showed no benefit when comparing simvastatin monotherapy to simvastatin/ezetimibe combination therapy in rates of progression of carotid intima media thickness in patients with heterozygous familial hypercholesterolemia. There are no endpoint trials either completed or underway which compare a statin to statin/bile acid binding resin or statin/fish oil therapies.

In high and very high risk patients, the primary goal of therapy is to lower LDL-C to NCEP goals, or a minimum of 30–40%. For many of these patients, this will require moderate to high dose statin therapy. Adjuvant lipid lowering therapy with niacin, fenofibrate, ezetimibe, or a bile acid binding resin can be used to help further adjust serum lipoprotein levels. The choice of adjuvant therapy is driven by the specifics of the lipid profile. In the absence of clinical endpoint data, combination therapy (with the exception of statin/niacin therapy) is currently used to further optimize the lipid profile. In the years ahead, the capacity of adjuvant lipid lowering therapy to augment risk reduction in a safe and tolerable manner when used in combination with a statin will be further defined. In the meantime, it is advisable to titrate a statin to the highest necessary dose in order to attain LDL-C goals. In patients with mixed dyslipidemia, consideration should be given to a statin's pharmacologic profile to not only lower LDL-C, but also reduce TG and raise HDL-C. If moderate to high dose statin therapy provides insufficient capacity to attain lipoprotein targets, then consideration can be given to the addition of other agents. In the setting of combination therapy, although risk for adverse events remains relatively low, appropriate monitoring for toxicity (hepatotoxicity, myopathy, drug interactions) should be performed. Careful attention should also be directed at the dosing recommendations in the package insert for each of the drugs used so as to minimize risk for adverse events.

REFERENCES

[1] Grundy, S.M. (2001) United States Cholesterol Guidelines 2001: expanded scope of intensive low-density lipoprotein-lowering therapy. *The American Journal of Cardiology*, **88**, 23J–27J.

[2] National Cholesterol Education Program, Expert Panel on Detection, Evaluation, and Treatment of High Blood Cholesterol in Adults (Adult Treatment Panel III) (2001) Executive summary of the third report of the National Cholesterol Education Program (NCEP). *The Journal of the American Medical Association*, **285**, 2486–97.

[3] Jones, P.H., Davidson, M.H., Stein, E.A. *et al.* (2003) Comparison of the efficacy and safety of rosuvastatin versus atorvastatin, simvastatin, and pravastatin across doses (STELLAR* Trial). *The American Journal of Cardiology*, **92**, 152–60.

[4] Jones, P., Kafonek, S., Laurora, I. and Hunninghake, D. (1998) Comparative dose efficacy study of atorvastatin versus simvastatin, pravastatin, lovastatin, and fluvastatin in patients with hypercholesterolemia (the CURVES study). *The American Journal of Cardiology*, **81**, 582–87.

[5] LaRosa, J.C., Grundy, S.M., Waters, D.D. *et al*. (2005) Intensive lipid lowering with atorvastatin in patients with stable coronary disease. *The New England Journal of Medicine*, **352**, 1425–35.

[6] Cannon, C.P., Braunwald, E., McCabe, C.H. *et al*. (2004) Intensive versus moderate lipid lowering with statins after acute coronary syndromes. *The New England Journal of Medicine*, **350**, 1495–504.

[7] Davidson, M.H. and Robinson, J.G. (2007) Safety of aggressive lipid management. *Journal of the American College of Cardiology*, **49**, 1753–62.

[8] Brown, B.G., Zhao, X.Q., Chait, A. *et al*. (2001) Simvastatin and niacin, antioxidant vitamins, or the combination for the prevention of coronary disease. *The New England Journal of Medicine*, **345**, 1583–92.

[9] Taylor, A.J., Sullenberger, L.E., Lee, H.J. *et al*. (2004) Arterial Biology for the Investigation of the Treatment Effects of Reducing Cholesterol (ARBITER) 2: a double-blind, placebo-controlled study of extended-release niacin on atherosclerosis progression in secondary prevention patients treated with statins. *Circulation*, **110**, 3512–17.

[10] Jones, P.H. and Davidson, M.H. (2005) Reporting rate of rhabdomyolysis with fenofibrate + statin versus gemfibrozil + any statin. *The American Journal of Cardiology*, **95**, 120–22.

[11] Davidson, M.H. and Toth, P.P. (2004) Comparative effects of lipid-lowering therapies. *Progress in Cardiovascular Diseases*, **47**, 73–104.

CONTROVERSY

DO THE BENEFITS OF LOW-DENSITY LIPOPROTEIN CHOLESTEROL REDUCTION DEPEND STRICTLY ON "HOW LOW YOU GO" OR ALSO ON "HOW YOU GET THERE"?

New Controversies Resulting from the ENHANCE (Ezetimibe and Simvastatin in Hypercholesterolemia Enhances Atherosclerosis Regression) Trial

Not long before this book was scheduled to go to press, results from the ENHANCE trial were released, producing a firestorm of debate among scientists and clinicians [1–3]. The controversy centers on the appropriateness of assuming that new agents that effectively lower LDL-C will reduce cardiovascular events in the absence of data from cardiovascular event trials. The prevailing view during the prior decade has been that the evidence showing benefits of LDL-C reduction through a variety of interventions (statin drugs, bile acid sequestrants, niacin, ileal bypass surgery, dietary intervention) was strong enough to warrant the view that the most important consideration was reaching treatment targets (i.e. how low you go) and not the type of therapy used to achieve those goals (i.e. how you get there).

Two types of compounds that lower LDL-C had previously failed to show benefits in clinical event trials: conjugated equine estrogens (with or without medroxyprogesterone acetate) and torcetrapib (a cholesteryl ester transfer protein inhibitor). However, these drugs also had identifiable off-target effects that might be reasonably expected to offset the benefits of LDL-C reductions. Conjugated estrogens also raise triglycerides and C-reactive protein (CRP), increase thrombogenicity and activate metalloproteinases that may destabilize atherosclerotic plaques [4–6]. Torcetrapib increases blood pressure, as well as serum aldosterone and bicarbonate levels and reduces circulating potassium [7].

In contrast, ezetimibe, the agent studied in ENHANCE, is minimally absorbed systemically and exerts its effects on the lipid profile through reducing intestinal absorption of cholesterol by binding the Nieman-Pick C1-like-1 protein in the intestinal wall. In addition to lowering LDL-C, ezetimibe reduces apolipoprotein (Apo) B, triglycerides and CRP. No off-target effects have been identified that would be expected to offset its favorable effects on the lipid profile.

In the ENHANCE trial 720 patients with heterozygous familial hypercholesterolemia were randomly assigned to receive 80 mg per day of simvastatin plus either ezetimibe 10 mg per day or placebo [3] for two years. The primary outcome variable was the change from baseline in intima-media thickness of the carotid artery (CIMT), a surrogate marker for progression of atherosclerosis. Despite significantly lower levels (all $p < 0.01$) of LDL-C (141 versus 193 mg dl^{-1}), Apo B (135 versus 169 mg dl^{-1}), triglycerides (108 versus 120 mg dl^{-1}) and CRP (0.9 versus 1.2 mg l^{-1}) during treatment, the group receiving ezetimibe showed a mean change in CIMT that was no different from that in the group receiving placebo (0.0111 versus 0.0058 mm, respectively in the ezetimibe and placebo groups, respectively, $p = 0.29$).

The lack of benefit of ezetimibe on CIMT was surprising since other trials have found that more aggressive treatment of hypercholesterolemia results in slowed progression or even regression of CIMT [8–11]. For example, the Atorvastatin versus Simvastatin on Atherosclerosis Progression (ASAP) trial studied a group of 325 subjects with heterozygous familial hypercholesterolemia [8]. The results showed that more aggressive lowering of LDL-C with 80 mg per day of atorvastatin produced regression of CIMT (−0.031 mm), while the group that received less aggressive statin therapy (40 mg per day of simvastatin) showed progression of 0.036 mm ($p = 0.0001$ for the comparison between groups).

Given that other studies using the same methods of measurement have shown benefits of more aggressive LDL-C therapy, at least two potential explanations exist for the lack of benefit associated with ezetimibe treatment during the ENHANCE trial:

1. Ezetimibe may not be antiatherogenic, despite its ability to lower LDL-C, atherogenic lipoprotein particles and CRP.
2. The participants in the ENHANCE trial may have had a lower than expected risk of progression, limiting the ability of the study to demonstrate a benefit.

Regarding the first issue, ezetimibe could have as yet unidentified off-target adverse effects. While this cannot be entirely ruled out, the fact that it is minimally absorbed reduces the likelihood that this is the explanation. Alternatively, ezetimibe may fail to provide some benefit that is obtained with the use of other agents. Ezetimibe does not generally raise HDL-C and in some studies has failed to improve endothelial function [12, 13]. However, a recent meta-regression study conducted by Robinson *et al.* [14] showed that the relationship between LDL-C lowering and the reduction in risk of coronary heart disease over five years of treatment was not dependent on the type of treatment that induced the LDL-C reduction. Thus, lowering LDL-C through the use of dietary intervention (5 studies), bile acid sequestrants (3 studies), ileal bypass (1 study) and statin therapy (10 studies) produced similar reductions in risk for a given reduction in LDL-C, arguing against a large influence of effects beyond those of reducing LDL-C and atherogenic lipoproteins. Data from imaging studies suggest that changes in both atherogenic (LDL-C) and antiatherogenic (HDL-C) lipoprotein cholesterol levels predict changes in atheroma volume [15]. Nevertheless, due to the generally greater effect of drug therapy on LDL-C, the influence of changes in LDL-C is quantitatively larger. Therefore, while it is possible that the lack of some benefit beyond the reduction in LDL-C and atherogenic lipoproteins accounts for the failure to demonstrate a benefit of treatment with ezetimibe, this also appears to be unlikely given the available evidence.

In the authors' view, the more likely explanation for the lack of difference in progression between treatments in the ENHANCE trial is the low baseline CIMT values in both treatment groups. In the ASAP trial, initial CIMT value was the strongest predictor of the degree of progression, with higher baseline CIMT associated with greater progression [9]. The subjects in the ENHANCE and ASAP trials were of similar age with the same underlying condition (familial hypercholesterolemia). Table 1 shows selected characteristics for the subjects assigned to the simvastatin monotherapy arms in the two studies. Before and during treatment the subjects in the two trials receiving simvastatin monotherapy had similar levels of LDL-C. However, the baseline CIMT in the ASAP trial was 31% larger (0.92 versus 0.70 mm). In fact, the baseline CIMT among ENHANCE trial participants was similar to the mean value among subjects without CHD in the Atherosclerosis Risk in Communities study (0.72 mm, 16). CIMT progression over two years among subjects in the ASAP trial receiving simvastatin monotherapy was six times that for subjects in ENHANCE trial receiving simvastatin monotherapy (0.0360 versus 0.0058 mm). Thus, despite receiving the same drug and having similar levels of LDL-C at baseline and during treatment, subjects in the simvastatin monotherapy arm in the ENHANCE trial had much lower baseline CIMT and only a fraction of the CIMT progression that was observed in the simvastatin monotherapy arm in the ASAP trial. The fact that the comparator arm in the ENHANCE trial showed essentially no CIMT progression suggests that the ability of an additional therapy to show incremental benefit may have been limited. This is analogous to conducting a cardiovascular event trial in children. No matter how effective the lipid alteration, one would not expect to find a difference between treatments in events since the event rate would be too low in both groups to demonstrate a benefit.

What might account for these different responses in the comparator arms of these two studies? One potential explanation is that usual care for management of familial hypercholesterolemia changed during the time between the ASAP and ENHANCE trials. Most ENHANCE trial participants had their lipid therapy stopped temporarily prior to the baseline lipid measurements. Subjects who participated in the ENHANCE trial were likely to have been treated more aggressively before entering the study because standards of care changed over the several years before recruitment began, favoring more aggressive therapy. Aggressive management of lipids and other risk factors over a period of several years before entering the trial may have produced changes in the carotid artery wall, rendering it less likely to respond to additional therapy. In fact, over the two-year extension to the ASAP trial, subjects who continued on 80 mg per day of atorvastatin had little additional change in CIMT (0.005 mm per year or 0.010 mm over two years). This is nearly identical to the degree of progression observed in the simvastatin plus ezetimibe group in the ENHANCE trial (0.011 mm). Thus, the failure to observe a difference between treatments in the ENHANCE trial may have been a case of an inability to "make healthy arteries healthier".

The panel convened to discuss the clinical implications of the ENHANCE trial at the American College of Cardiology meeting, as well as the two editorials in the *New England Journal of Medicine* that accompanied the ENHANCE paper recommended that, in light of the failure to show a benefit of adding ezetimibe to simvastatin in the ENHANCE trial, ezetimibe should be reserved for use in patients who cannot tolerate other drug classes or who cannot achieve their treatment targets with statins plus niacin, fibrates or bile acid sequestrants. At the American College of Cardiology meeting, there was no meaningful debate about the validity of the results or the design of the study. Many physicians in attendance disagreed with both the content and tone of the discussants' presentation. Press coverage also appeared heavily weighted toward the extraordinarily negative opinions of a few physicians. The press even managed to call the entire "LDL hypothesis" into question, resulting in considerable confusion among patients, many of whom discontinued their therapy based on newspaper and television reports. This constitutes a profound disservice to patients. Physicians also began to withdraw patients from ezetimibe therapy out of fear that continuing the drug would leave them exposed to litigation.

Ezetimibe accounted for more than 15% of the total prescriptions for lipid therapy in the United States in 2006 [17]. Therefore, moving it to the "back of the line" would have substantial implications for lipid management. Ezetimibe has been popular because of its favorable safety and side effect profiles, as well as its efficacy for lowering LDL-C, particularly as an adjunct to a statin. Its use significantly increases the number of high and very high risk patients able to attain their LDL-C goals [18–23].

The authors of this book disagree with the conclusion that ezetimibe should be moved to the back of the line as a treatment for dyslipidemia. We are of the opinion that the atherogenicity of Apo B-containing lipoproteins has been well enough established that, in the absence of a compelling reason to believe that off-target adverse effects may be at work, the demonstrated effects on atherogenic lipoproteins are sufficient to tip the odds in favor of a presumed net benefit. Achieving the newer optional treatment targets for LDL-C and non-HDL-C is difficult without combination therapy in many patients. For most, statin therapy will be the first line of drug therapy. Of the available treatment options, we only have direct evidence of benefit with addition to a statin for niacin [24]. The combination niacin and simvastatin has been shown to be effective for reducing the progression of coronary atherosclerosis and CIMT [25, 26]. No large scale outcome trials have been completed for combinations of lipid drug therapies.

The recently published Stop Atherosclerosis in Native Diabetics Study (SANDS) illustrated the difficulty of achieving more aggressive treatment goals. In this trial [27], 499 Native American subjects with type 2 diabetes (but free of clinical CHD), were assigned to receive standard care for lipids and blood pressure (LDL-C goal $<100\,\mathrm{mg\ dl^{-1}}$ and systolic blood pressure goal $<130\,\mathrm{mm\ Hg}$) or aggressive treatment (LDL-C goal $<70\,\mathrm{mg\ dl^{-1}}$ and systolic blood pressure goal $<115\,\mathrm{mm\ Hg}$) for three years. The surrogate markers of CIMT and left ventricular mass were the main outcome variables. Among patients unable to reach their LDL-C target in this trial, ezetimibe was added. Aggressive LDL-C and blood pressure reduction resulted in significant improvements in CIMT and left ventricular mass. Mean on-treatment levels of LDL-C ($72\,\mathrm{mg\ dl^{-1}}$) and systolic blood pressure ($117\,\mathrm{mm\ Hg}$) in the aggressive treatment arm indicate that fewer than half of subjects were able to achieve and maintain the treatment goals, even in the setting of a clinical trial. The authors believe that the net impact of a recommendation to move ezetimibe to the back of the line as a lipid treatment will likely result in fewer patients reaching their treatment targets. While we feel that the best evidence to guide clinical decisions arises from randomized clinical event trials, such data for ezetimibe will not be available before 2011 at the earliest (from the ongoing IMPROVE-IT or Improved Reduction of Outcomes: VYTORIN Efficacy International Trial) and no such data are available for combinations of statin therapy with any other lipid altering drug. In the meantime, for the reasons cited above, our view is that the ENHANCE trial does not raise sufficient doubts about the likelihood of benefit with ezetimibe to warrant any change in clinical practice[1]. This is consistent with a position statement released by the National Lipid Association released in January of 2008 [28].

REFERENCES

[1] Brown, B.G. and Taylor, A.J. (2008) Does ENHANCE diminish confidence in lowering LDL or in ezetimibe. *The New England Journal of Medicine*, **358**, 1504–6.
[2] Drazen, J.M., Jarcho, J.A., Morissey, S. and Curfman, G.D. (2008) Cholesterol lowering and ezetimibe. *The New England Journal of Medicine*, **358**, 1507–8.
[3] Kastelein, J.J.P., Akdim, F., Stroes, E.S.G. *et al.* (2008) Simvastatin with or without ezetimibe in familial hypercholesterolemia. *The New England Journal of Medicine*, **358**, 1431–43.
[4] Luyer, M.D.P., Khosla, S., Owen, W.G. and Miller, V.M. (2001) Prospective randomized study of effects of unopposed estrogen replacement therapy on markers of coagulation and inflammation in postmenopausal women. *The Journal of Clinical Endocrinology and Metabolism*, **86**, 3629–34.
[5] Koh, K.K., Shin, M-S., Sakuma, I. *et al.* (2004) Effects of conventional or lower doses of hormone replacement therapy in postmenopausal women. *Arteriosclerosis, Thrombosis, and Vascular Biology*, **24**, 1516–21.
[6] Lewandowski, K.C., Komorowski, J., Mikhalidis, D.P. *et al.* (2006) Effects of hormone replacement therapy type and route of administration on plasma matrix metalloproteinases and their tissue inhibitors in postmenopausal women. *The Journal of Clinical Endocrinology and Metabolism*, **91**, 3123–30.
[7] Barter, P.J., Caulfield, M., Eriksson, M. *et al.* (2007) Effects of torcetrapib in patients at high risk for coronary events. *The New England Journal of Medicine*, **357**, 2109–22.
[8] Smilde, T.J., van Wissen, S., Wollersheim, H. *et al.* (2001) Effect of aggressive versus conventional lipid lowering on atherosclerosis progression in familial hypercholesterolemia (ASAP): a prospective, randomized, double-blind trial. *Lancet*, **357**, 577–81.
[9] Van Wissen, S., Smilde, T.J., Trip, M.D. *et al.* (2005) Long-term safety and efficacy of high-dose atorvastatin treatment in patients with familial hypercholesterolemia. *The American Journal of Cardiology*, **95**, 264–66.

[1]The authors wish to disclose that both have received support in the form of research grants and/or consulting fees/honoraria from the manufacturers of ezetimibe (Merck/Schering Plough).

[10] Nissen, S.E., Nicholls, S.J., Sipahi, I. *et al*. ATSERIOD Investigators. (2006) Effect of very-high intensity statin therapy on regression of coronary atherosclerosis: the ASTEROID trial. *The Journal of the American Medical Association*, **295**, 1556–65.

[11] Crouse J.R. III, Raichlen J.S., Riley W.A. *et al*. (2007) Effect of rosuvastatin on progression of carotid intima-media thickness in low-risk individuals with subclinical atherosclerosis: The METEOR Trial. *The Journal of the American Medical Association*, **297**, 1344–53.

[12] Landmesser, U., Bahlmann, F., Mueller, M. *et al*. (2005) Simvastatin versus ezetimibe: pleiotropic and lipid-lowering effects on endothelial function in humans. *Circulation*, **111**, 2356–63.

[13] Fichtischerer, S., Schmidt-Lucke, C., Bojunga, S. *et al*. (2006) Differential effects of short-term lipid lowering with ezetimibe and statins on endothelial function in patients with CAD; clinical evidence for "pleiotropic" functions of statin therapy. *European Heart Journal*, **27**, 1182–90.

[14] Robinson, J.G., Smith, B., Maheshwari, N. and Schrott, H. (2005) Pleiotropic effects of statins: benefit beyond cholesterol reduction? A meta-regression analysis. *Journal of the American College of Cardiology*, **46**, 1855–62.

[15] Nicholls, S.J., Tuzcu, E.M., Sipahi, I. *et al*. (2007) Statins, high-density lipoprotein cholesterol, and regression of coronary atherosclerosis. *The Journal of the American Medical Association*, **297**, 499–508.

[16] Chambless, L.E., Heiss, G., Folsom, A.R. *et al*. (1997) Association of coronary heart disease incidence with carotid arterial wall thickness and major risk factors: The Atherosclerosis Risk in Communities (ARIC) Study, 1987–1993. *American Journal of Epidemiology*, **146**, 483–94.

[17] Jackevicius, C.A., Tu, J.V., Ross, J.S. *et al*. (2008) Use of ezetimibe in the United States and Canada. *The New England Journal of Medicine*, **358**, 1819–28.

[18] Knopp, R.H., Gitter, H., Truitt, T. *et al*. (2003) Effects of ezetimibe, a new cholesterol absorption inhibitor, on plasma lipids in patients with primary hypercholesterolemia. *European Heart Journal*, **24**, 729–41.

[19] Abate, N., Catapano, A.L., Ballantyne, C.M. and Davidson, M.H. (2008) Effect of ezetimibe/simvastain versus atorvastatin or rosuvastatin on modifying lipid profiles in patients with diabetes, metabolic syndrome, or neither: results of two subgroup analyses. *Journal of Clinical Lipidology*, **2**, 91–105.

[20] Davidson, M.H., Ballantyne, C.M., Kerzner, B. *et al*. (2006) Effectiveness of ezetimibe added to ongoing statin therapy in modifying lipid profiles and low-density lipoprotein cholesterol goal attainment in patients of different races and ethnicities: a substudy of the Ezetimibe add-on to statin for effectiveness trial. *Mayo Clinic Proceedings*, **81**, 1177–85.

[21] Denke, M., Pearson, T., McBride, P. *et al.* (2006) Ezetimibe added to ongoing statin therapy improves LDL-C goal attainment and lipid profile in patients with diabetes or metabolic syndrome. *Diabetes and Vascular Disease Research*, **3**, 93–102.

[22] Guyton, J.R., Goldberg, R.B., Mazzone, T. *et al.* (2008) Lipoprotein and apolipoprotein ratios in the VYTAL trial of ezetimibe/simvastatin compared with atorvastatin in type 2 diabetes. *Journal of Clinical Lipidology*, **2**, 19–24.

[23] Pearson, T.A., Denke, M.A., McBride, P.E. *et al.* (2006) Effectiveness of ezetimibe added to ongoing statin therapy in modifying lipid profiles and low-density lipoprotein cholesterol goal attainment in patients of different races and ethnicities: a substudy of the Ezetimibe add-on to statin for effectiveness trial. *Mayo Clinic Proceedings*, **81**, 1177–85.

[24] Ballantyne, C.M., Davidson, M.H., McKenney, J. *et al.* (2008) Comparison of the safety and efficacy of a combination tablet niacin extended release and simvastatin vs. simvastatin monotherapy in patients with increased non-HDL cholesterol (from the SEACOAST I Study). *The American Journal of Cardiology*, **101**, 1428–36.

[25] Taylor, A.J., Lee, H.J., Sullenberger, L.E. (2006) The effect of 24 months of combination statin and extended-release niacin on carotid intima-media thickness. ARBITER 3. *Current Medical Research and Opinion*, **22**, 2243–50.

[26] Taylor, A.J., Sullenberger, L.E., Lee, H.J. *et al.* (2004) Arterial Biology for the Investigation of the Treatment Effects of Reducing Cholesterol (ARBITER) 2: a double-blind, placebo-controlled study of extended-release niacin on atherosclerosis progression in secondary prevention patients treated with statins. *Circulation*, **110**, 3512–17.

[27] Howard, B.V., Roman, M.J., Devereux, R.B. *et al.* (2008) Effect of lower targets for blood pressure and LDL cholesterol on atherosclerosis in diabetes: The SANDS randomized trial. *The Journal of the American Medical Association*, **299**, 1678–89.

[28] National Lipid Association. (2008) Statement on ENHANCE study findings: premature judgment unwarranted. Accessed 5/19/08 at http://www.lipid.org/press/index.php.

REFERENCES

[1] Rosamond, W., Flegal, K., Friday, G. *et al.* (2007) Heart disease and stroke statistics – 2007 update: a report from the American Heart Association Statistics Committee and Stroke Statistics Subcommittee. *Circulation*, **115**, e69–e171.

[2] Grundy, S.M., Cleeman, J.I., Merz, C.N. *et al.* Coordinating Committee of the National Cholesterol Education Program (2004) Implications of recent clinical trials for the National Cholesterol Education Program Adult Treatment Panel III Guidelines. [Review] [45 refs]. *Journal of the American College of Cardiology*, **44**, 720–32.

[3] Baigent, C., Keech, A., Kearney, P.M. *et al.* (2005) Efficacy and safety of cholesterol-lowering treatment: prospective meta-analysis of data from 90,056 participants in 14 randomised trials of statins. [see comment] [erratum appears in (2005) Lancet, 366(9494), 1358]. *Lancet*, **366**, 1267–78.

[4] National Cholesterol Education Program Expert Panel on Detection EaTo-HBCiA (2002) Third report of the National Cholesterol Education Program (NCEP) Expert Panel on Detection, Evaluation, and Treatment of High Blood Cholesterol in Adults (Adult Treatment Panel III) final report. [see comment]. *Circulation*, **106**, 3143–421.

[5] Wilson, P.W., D'Agostino, R.B., Levy, D. *et al.* (1998) Prediction of coronary heart disease using risk factor categories. [see comment]. *Circulation*, **97**, 1837–47.

[6] Stamler, J., Wentworth, D. and Neaton, J.D. (1986) Is relationship between serum cholesterol and risk of premature death from coronary heart disease continuous and graded? Findings in 356,222 primary screenees of the Multiple Risk Factor Intervention Trial (MRFIT). *The Journal of the American Medical Association*, **256**, 2823–28.

[7] *The Journal of the American Medical Association* (1984) The lipid research clinics coronary primary prevention trial results. I. Reduction in incidence of coronary heart disease, **251**, 351–64.

[8] Verschuren, W.M., Jacobs, D.R., Bloemberg, B.P. *et al.* (1995) Serum total cholesterol and long-term coronary heart disease mortality in different cultures. Twenty-five-year follow-up of the seven countries study. *The Journal of the American Medical Association*, **274**, 131–36.

[9] Yusuf, S., Hawken, S., Ounpuu, S. *et al.* (2004) Effect of potentially modifiable risk factors associated with myocardial infarction in 52 countries (the INTERHEART study): case-control study. *Lancet*, **364**, 937–52.

[10] Steyn, K., Sliwa, K., Hawken, S. *et al.* (2005) Risk factors associated with myocardial infarction in Africa: the INTERHEART Africa study. *Circulation*, **112**, 3554–61.

[11] *The Journal of the American Medical Association* (1984) The lipid research clinics coronary primary prevention trial results. II. The relationship of reduction in incidence of coronary heart disease to cholesterol lowering. **251**, 365–74.

[12] Pedersen, T.R., Olsson, A.G., Faergeman, O. *et al.* (1998) Lipoprotein changes and reduction in the incidence of major coronary heart disease events in the Scandinavian Simvastatin Survival Study (4S) [see comment]. *Circulation*, **97**, 1453–60.

[13] Robinson, J.G., Smith, B., Maheshwari, N. and Schrott, H. (2005) Pleiotropic effects of statins: benefit beyond cholesterol reduction? A meta-regression analysis. [see comment]. *Journal of the American College of Cardiology*, **46**, 1855–62.

[14] Grundy, S.M., Cleeman, J.I., Merz, C.N. *et al.* (2004) Implications of recent clinical trials for the National Cholesterol Education Program Adult Treatment Panel III guidelines. *Circulation*, **110**, 227–39.

[15] Sarnak, M.J., Levey, A.S., Schoolwerth, A.C. *et al.* (2003) Kidney disease as a risk factor for development of cardiovascular disease: a statement from the American Heart Association Councils on Kidney in Cardiovascular Disease, High Blood Pressure Research, Clinical Cardiology, and Epidemiology and Prevention. *Circulation*, **108**, 2154–69.

100   LOW-DENSITY LIPOPROTEIN CHOLESTEROL

[16] Toth, P. (2007) Intensive LDL-C lowering: which patients benefit. *Family Practice Recertification*, **29**, 24–37.
[17] Toth, P. (2007) Why do patients at highest CV risk receive the least treatment? The danger of doing too little. *Resident and Staff Physician*, **53**, s1–s7.
[18] LaRosa, J.C., Grundy, S.M., Waters, D.D. *et al.* (2005) Intensive lipid lowering with atorvastatin in patients with stable coronary disease. [see comment]. *The New England Journal of Medicine*, **352**, 1425–35.
[19] Cannon, C.P., Braunwald, E., McCabe, C.H. *et al.* (2004) Intensive versus moderate lipid lowering with statins after acute coronary syndromes. [see comment] [erratum appears in (2006) New England Journal of Medicine, 354(7), 778]. *The New England Journal of Medicine*, **350**, 1495–504.
[20] Whitney, E. (1999) The Air Force/Texas Coronary Atherosclerosis Prevention Study: Implications for Preventive Cardiology in the General Adult US Population. *Current Atherosclerosis Reports*, **1**, 38–43.
[21] Sever, P.S., Dahlof, B., Poulter, N.R. *et al.* (2003) Prevention of coronary and stroke events with atorvastatin in hypertensive patients who have average or lower-than-average cholesterol concentrations, in the Anglo-Scandinavian Cardiac Outcomes Trial–Lipid Lowering Arm (ASCOT-LLA): a multicentre randomised controlled trial. [see comment]. *Lancet*, **361**, 1149–58.
[22] Colhoun, H.M., Betteridge, D.J., Durrington, P.N. *et al.* (2004) Primary prevention of cardiovascular disease with atorvastatin in type 2 diabetes in the Collaborative Atorvastatin Diabetes Study (CARDS): multicentre randomised placebo-controlled trial. [see comment]. *Lancet*, **364**, 685–96.
[23] Heart Protection Study Collaborative Group (2002) MRC/BHF Heart Protection Study of cholesterol lowering with simvastatin in 20, 536 high-risk individuals: a randomised placebo-controlled trial. [see comment] [summary for patients in (2002) Current cardiology reports, 4(6), 486–7, PMID: 12379169]. *Lancet*, **360**, 7–22.
[24] Shepherd, J., Blauw, G.J., Murphy, M.B. *et al.* (2002) Pravastatin in elderly individuals at risk of vascular disease (PROSPER): a randomised controlled trial. [see comment]. *Lancet*, **360**, 1623–30.
[25] Shepherd, J., Cobbe, S.M., Ford, I. *et al.* (1995) Prevention of coronary heart disease with pravastatin in men with hypercholesterolemia. West of Scotland Coronary Prevention Study Group. [see comment]. *The New England Journal of Medicine*, **333**, 1301–7.
[26] Scandinavian Simvastatin Survival Study Group (1994) Randomised trial of cholesterol lowering in 4444 patients with coronary heart disease: the Scandinavian Simvastatin Survival Study (4S). *Lancet*, **344**, 1383–89.
[27] Pitt, B., Waters, D., Brown, W.V. Atorvastatin versus Revascularization Treatment Investigators (1999) Aggressive lipid-lowering therapy compared with angioplasty in stable coronary artery disease. *The New England Journal of Medicine*, **341**, 70–76.
[28] Sacks, F.M., Pfeffer, M.A., Moye, L.A. *et al.* (1996) The effect of pravastatin on coronary events after myocardial infarction in patients with average cholesterol levels. Cholesterol and Recurrent Events Trial investigators. [see comment]. *The New England Journal of Medicine*, **335**, 1001–9.
[29] The LIPID Study Group (1995) Design features and baseline characteristics of the LIPID (Long-Term Intervention with Pravastatin in Ischemic Disease)

Study: a randomized trial in patients with previous acute myocardial infarction and/or unstable angina pectoris. *The American Journal of Cardiology*, **76**, 474–79.

[30] Serruys, P.W., de Feyter, P., Macaya, C. *et al.* (2002) Fluvastatin for prevention of cardiac events following successful first percutaneous coronary intervention. A randomized controlled trial. *The Journal of the American Medical Association*, **287**, 3215–22.

[31] Schwartz, G.G., Olsson, A.G., Ezekowitz, M.D. *et al.* (2001) Effects of atorvastatin on early recurrent ischemic events in acute coronary syndromes: the MIRACL study: a randomized controlled trial. *The Journal of the American Medical Association*, **285**, 1711–18.

[32] Nissen, S. (2004) Aggressive lipid-lowering therapy and regression of coronary atheroma. *The Journal of the American Medical Association*, **292**, 1–3.

[33] Toth, P.P. and Davidson, M.H. (2005) Simvastatin plus ezetimibe: combination therapy for the management of dyslipidaemia. *Expert Opinion on Pharmacotherapy*, **6**, 131–39.

[34] Schaefer, E.J., Genest, J.J., Ordovas, J.M. *et al.* (1994) Familial lipoprotein disorders and premature coronary artery disease. *Atherosclerosis*, **108**, S41–S54.

[35] Davidson, M.H. and Robinson, J.R. (2007) Management of Elevated Low-Density Lipoprotein Cholesterol, in *Comprehensive Management of High Risk Cardiovascular Patients*, (eds A.M. Gotto and P.P. Toth), Informa Pub, New York, pp. 255–93.

[36] Grundy, S.M. (1997) Small LDL, atherogenic dyslipidemia, and the metabolic syndrome. [comment]. *Circulation*, **95**, 1–4.

[37] Toth, P.P. (2004) Low-density lipoprotein reduction in high-risk patients: how low do you go? *Current Atherosclerosis Reports*, **6**, 348–52.

[38] Krauss, R.M. (2005) Dietary and genetic probes of atherogenic dyslipidemia. *Arteriosclerosis, Thrombosis and Vascular Biology*, **25**, 2265–72.

[39] Lamarche, B., Tchernof, A., Moorjani, S. *et al.* (1997) Small, dense low-density lipoprotein particles as a predictor of the risk of ischemic heart disease in men. Prospective results from the Quebec Cardiovascular Study. [see comment]. *Circulation*, **95**, 69–75.

[40] Blake, G.J., Otvos, J.D., Rifai, N. and Ridker, P.M. (2002) Low-density lipoprotein particle concentration and size as determined by nuclear magnetic resonance spectroscopy as predictors of cardiovascular disease in women. *Circulation*, **106**, 1930–37.

[41] Kuller, L., Arnold, A., Tracy, R. *et al.* (2002) Nuclear magnetic resonance spectroscopy of lipoproteins and risk of coronary heart disease in the cardiovascular health study. *Arteriosclerosis, Thrombosis, and Vascular Biology*, **22**, 1175–80.

[42] Kathiresan, S., Otvos, J.D., Sullivan, L.M. *et al.* (2006) Increased small low-density lipoprotein particle number: a prominent feature of the metabolic syndrome in the Framingham Heart Study. *Circulation*, **113**, 20–29.

[43] Otvos, J.D., Collins, D., Freedman, D.S. *et al.* (2006) Low-density lipoprotein and high-density lipoprotein particle subclasses predict coronary events and are favorably changed by gemfibrozil therapy in the Veterans Affairs High-Density Lipoprotein Intervention Trial. *Circulation*, **113**, 1556–63.

[44] Schwartz, C.J., Valente, A.J. and Sprague, E.A. (1993) A modern view of atherogenesis. *The American Journal of Cardiology*, **71**, 25.

[45] Brown, M.S. and Goldstein, J.L. (1986) A receptor-mediated pathway for cholesterol homeostasis. *Science*, **232**, 34–47.

[46] Hobbs, H.H., Russell, D.W., Brown, M.S. and Goldstein, J.L. (1990) The LDL receptor locus in familial hypercholesterolemia: mutational analysis of a membrane protein. *Annual Review of Genetics*, **24**, 133–70.

[47] van Aalst-Cohen, E.S., Jansen, A.C., de Jongh, S. *et al.* (2004) Clinical, diagnostic, and therapeutic aspects of familial hypercholesterolemia. *Seminars in Vascular Medicine*, **4**, 31–41.

[48] Moriarty, P.M. (2006) LDL-apheresis Therapy. *Current Treatment Options in Cardiovascular Medicine*, **8**, 282–88.

[49] Toth, P. (2006) *Dyslipoproteinemias*, W.B. Saunders, Philadelphia.

[50] Martin, G., Duez, H., Blanquart, C. *et al.* (2001) Statin-induced inhibition of the Rho-signaling pathway activates PPARalpha and induces HDL apoA-I. *The Journal of Clinical Investigation*, **107**, 1423–32.

[51] Liao, J.K. and Laufs, U. (2005) Pleiotropic effects of statins. *Annual Review of Pharmacology and Toxicology*, **45**, 89–118.

[52] Davidson, M.H. and Toth, P.P. (2004) Comparative effects of lipid-lowering therapies. *Progress in Cardiovascular Diseases*, **47**, 73–104.

[53] Nissen, S.E., Nicholls, S.J., Sipahi, I. *et al.* (2006) Effect of very high-intensity statin therapy on regression of coronary atherosclerosis: the ASTEROID trial. [see comment]. *The Journal of the American Medical Association*, **295**, 1556–65.

[54] Takemoto, M. and Liao, J.K. (2001) Pleiotropic effects of 3-hydroxy-3-methylglutaryl coenzyme a reductase inhibitors. *Arteriosclerosis, Thrombosis, and Vascular Biology*, **21**, 1712–19.

[55] Downs, J.R., Clearfield, M., Weis, S. *et al.* (1998) Primary prevention of acute coronary events with lovastatin in men and women with average cholesterol levels: results of AFCAPS/TexCAPS. Air Force/Texas Coronary Atherosclerosis Prevention Study. [see comment]. *The Journal of the American Medical Association*, **279**, 1615–22.

[56] *The New England Journal of Medicine* (1998) Prevention of cardiovascular events and death with pravastatin in patients with coronary heart disease and a broad range of initial cholesterol levels. The Long-Term Intervention with Pravastatin in Ischaemic Disease (LIPID) Study Group. [see comment]. **339**, 1349–57.

[57] Cannon, C.P., Steinberg, B.A., Murphy, S.A. *et al.* (2006) Meta-analysis of cardiovascular outcomes trials comparing intensive versus moderate statin therapy. *Journal of the American College of Cardiology*, **48**, 438–45.

[58] de Lemos, J.A., Blazing, M.A., Wiviott, S.D. *et al.* (2004) Early intensive vs a delayed conservative simvastatin strategy in patients with acute coronary syndromes: phase Z of the A to Z trial. [see comment]. *The Journal of the American Medical Association*, **292**, 1307–16.

[59] Pedersen, T.R., Faergeman, O., Kastelein, J.J. *et al.* (2005) High-dose atorvastatin vs usual-dose simvastatin for secondary prevention after myocardial infarction: the IDEAL study: a randomized controlled trial. [see comment][erratum appears in (2005) JAMA, 294(24), 3092] [reprint in (2006) Ugeskr Laeger,

168(18), 1769–71; PMID: 16729930]. *The Journal of the American Medical Association*, **294**, 2437–45.

[60] Toth, P.P. and Davidson, M.H. (2005) Cholesterol absorption blockade with ezetimibe. *Current Drug Targets. Cardiovascular and Haematological Disorders*, **5**, 455–62.

[61] Davis, H.R., Compton, D.S., Hoos, L. *et al.* (2000) Ezetimibe (SCH58235) localizes to the brush border to a small intestinal enterocyte and inhibits enterocyte cholesterol uptake and absorption. *European Heart Journal*, **21**(Suppl), 636.

[62] Catapano, A. (2001) Ezetimibe: a selective inhibitor of cholesterol absorption. *European Heart Journal*, **3** (Suppl E), E6–E10.

[63] Knopp, R.H., Bays, H., Manion, C.V. *et al.* (2001) Effect of ezetimibe on serum concentrations of lipid-soluble vitamins. *Atherosclerosis*, **2**, 90.

[64] Van Heek, M., France, C.F., Compton, D.S. *et al.* (1997) In vivo metabolism-based discovery of a potent cholesterol absorption inhibitor, SCH58235, in the rat and rhesus monkey through the identification of the active metabolites of SCH48461. *The Journal of Pharmacology and Experimental Therapeutics*, **283**, 157–63.

[65] Bays, H.E., Moore, P.B., Drehobl, M.A. *et al.* (2001) Effectiveness and tolerability of ezetimibe in patients with primary hypercholesterolemia: pooled analysis of two phase II studies. [erratum appears in (2001) Clinical Therapeutics, 23(9), 1601]. *Clinical Therapeutics*, **23**, 1209–30.

[66] Punwani, N., Pai, S., Bach, C. *et al.* (1998) Effect of food on oral bioavailability of SCH58235 in healthy male volunteers. *AAPS Pharmaceutical Sciences*, **1**, S486.

[67] Dujovne, C.A., Ettinger, M.P., McNeer, J.F. *et al.* Ezetimibe Study Group (2002) Efficacy and safety of a potent new selective cholesterol absorption inhibitor, ezetimibe, in patients with primary hypercholesterolemia. [erratum appears in (2003) The American Journal of Cardiology, 91(11), 1399]. *The American Journal of Cardiology*, **90**, 1092–97.

[68] Knopp, R.H., Gitter, H., Truitt, T. *et al.* (2003) Effects of ezetimibe, a new cholesterol absorption inhibitor, on plasma lipids in patients with primary hypercholesterolemia. *European Heart Journal*, **24**, 729–41.

[69] Davidson, M.H., McGarry, T., Bettis, R. *et al.* (2002) Ezetimibe coadministered with simvastatin in patients with primary hypercholesterolemia. [see comment]. *Journal of the American College of Cardiology*, **40**, 2125–34.

[70] Ballantyne, C.M., Houri, J., Notarbartolo, A. *et al.* (2003) Effect of ezetimibe coadministered with atorvastatin in 628 patients with primary hypercholesterolemia. *Circulation*, **19**, e9043–44.

[71] Kerzner, B., Corbelli, J., Sharp, S. *et al.* Ezetimibe Study Group (2003) Efficacy and safety of ezetimibe coadministered with lovastatin in primary hypercholesterolemia. *The American Journal of Cardiology*, **91**, 418–24.

[72] Melani, L., Mills, R., Hassman, D. *et al.* Ezetimibe Study Group (2003) Efficacy and safety of ezetimibe coadministered with pravastatin in patients with primary hypercholesterolemia: a prospective, randomized, double-blind trial. [see comment]. *European Heart Journal*, **24**, 717–28.

[73] Berge, K.E., Tian, H., Graf, G.A. *et al.* (2000) Accumulation of dietary cholesterol in sitosterolemia caused by mutations in adjacent ABC transporters. *Science*, **290**, 1771–75.

[74] Armani, A. and Toth, P.P. (2006) Colesevelam hydrochloride in the management of dyslipidemia. *Expert Review of Cardiovascular Therapy*, **4**, 283–91.

[75] Einarsson, K., Ericsson, S., Ewerth, S. *et al.* (1991) Bile acid sequestrants: mechanisms of action on bile acid and cholesterol metabolism. *European Journal of Clinical Pharmacology*, **40**, S53–S58.

[76] Davidson, M.H., Toth, P., Weiss, S. *et al.* (2001) Low-dose combination therapy with colesevelam hydrochloride and lovastatin effectively decreases low-density lipoprotein cholesterol in patients with primary hypercholesterolemia. *Clinical Cardiology*, **24**, 467–74.

[77] Knapp, H.H., Schrott, H., Ma, P. *et al.* (2001) Efficacy and safety of combination simvastatin and colesevelam in patients with primary hypercholesterolemia. *American Journal of Medicine*, **110**, 352–60.

[78] Hunninghake, D. Jr, Insull, W., Toth, P. *et al.* (2001) Coadministration of colesevelam hydrochloride with atorvastatin lowers LDL cholesterol additively. *Atherosclerosis*, **158**, 407–16.

[79] Insull, W. Jr (2006) Clinical utility of bile acid sequestrants in the treatment of dyslipidemia: a scientific review. *Southern Medical Journal*, **99**, 257–73.

[80] Steinmetz, K.L. and Schonder, K.S. (2005) Colesevelam: potential uses for the newest bile resin. *Cardiovascular Drug Reviews*, **23**, 15–30.

[81] McKenney, J.M., Davidson, M.H., Jacobson, T.A. and Guyton, J.R. National Lipid Association Statin Safety Assessment Task Force (2006) Final conclusions and recommendations of the National Lipid Association Statin Safety Assessment Task Force. *The American Journal of Cardiology*, **97**, 17.

[82] Pasternak, R.C., Smith, S.C. Jr, Bairey-Merz, C.N. *et al.* (2002) American College of Cardiology, American Heart Association, National Heart LaBI: ACC/AHA/NHLBI Clinical Advisory on the Use and Safety of Statins. [see comment]. *Stroke*, **33**, 2337–41.

[83] Marcoff, L. and Thompson, P.D. (2007) The role of coenzyme Q10 in statin-associated myopathy: a systematic review. *Journal of the American College of Cardiology*, **49**, 2231–37.

[84] Harper, C.R. and Jacobson, T.A. (2007) The broad spectrum of statin myopathy: from myalgia to rhabdomyolysis. *Current Opinion in Lipidology*, **18**, 401–8.

[85] Hanai, J.I., Cao, P., Tanksale, P. *et al.* (2007) The muscle-specific ubiquitin ligase atrogin-1/MAFbx mediates statin-induced muscle toxicity. *The Journal of Clinical Investigation*, **117**, 3940–51.

[86] Needham, M., Fabian, V., Knezevic, W. *et al.* (2007) Progressive myopathy with up-regulation of MHC-I associated with statin therapy. *Neuromuscular Disorders*, **17**, 194–200.

6 Management of Elevated Triglycerides and Non-high-density Lipoprotein Cholesterol

Key Points

- *The primary goal of lipid management is to achieve the patient's low-density lipoprotein cholesterol (LDL-C) treatment goal, but if the triglycerides (TG) concentration is still ≥ 200 mg dl^{-1}, non-high-density lipoprotein cholesterol (non-HDL-C) becomes a secondary target for intervention.*

- *Intensification of lifestyle modification, particularly weight loss and increased physical activity and smoking cessation, will reduce the underlying insulin resistance that is often associated with elevated TGs and can improve the lipid profile.*

- *For patients in whom lifestyle therapy is not sufficient to achieve the non-HDL-C treatment goal appropriate for the person's risk category (non-HDL-C goals are 30 mg dl^{-1} above the corresponding LDL-C goals), the non-HDL-C goal may be met by intensifying efforts to lower LDL-C or using interventions that target a reduction in very-low-density lipoprotein cholesterol (VLDL-C).*

- *Additional LDL-C lowering can be accomplished by adding or increasing the dose of statin therapy, adding plant sterols/stanols and viscous dietary fibers to the diet, or use of a cholesterol absorption inhibitor.*

- *Agents that primarily act to lower VLDL-C include fibrates, niacin, and omega-3 fatty acids.*

Practical Lipid Management: Concepts and Controversies   Peter P. Toth and Kevin C. Maki
© 2008 John Wiley & Sons, Ltd

As covered in detail in Chapter 3, the Adult Treatment Panel (ATP III) has adopted the following classification system for serum triglyceride (TG) levels:

- Normal TGs: <150 mg dl^{-1}
- Borderline-high TGs: 150–199 mg dl^{-1}
- High TGs: 200–499 mg dl^{-1}
- Very high TGs: ≥500 mg dl^{-1}

For patients with very high TGs, the initial goal of therapy is to reduce the TG concentration to below 500 mg dl^{-1} in order to prevent acute pancreatitis. For all other hypertriglyceridemic patients, cardiovascular risk reduction is the central focus. The National Cholesterol Education Panel Third Adult Treatment Panel (NCEP ATP III) recognized the greater strength of evidence linking TG-rich lipoproteins with atherosclerosis and coronary heart disease (CHD) event risk than was available at the time of the report of the ATP II. This led the panel to establish non-HDL-C goals that are 30 mg dl^{-1} higher than the corresponding LDL-C goals for the patient's risk category.

Non-HDL-C is a secondary therapeutic target (LDL-C is the primary target) for patients with TG ≥200 mg dl^{-1}. Thus, the treatment goals for non-HDL-C are <130, <160, and <190 mg dl^{-1} for patients with CHD or risk equivalents, multiple (≥2) major CHD risk factors, and 0–1 major CHD risk factors, respectively [1]. Optional non-HDL-C treatment targets for patients at very high risk (<100 mg dl^{-1}) and moderately high risk (<130 mg dl^{-1}) have also been recommended [2].

In clinical practice, encountering patients with elevated levels of TG and non-HDL-C is common. In the National Cholesterol Education Program Evaluation Project Utilizing Novel E-technology (NEPTUNE II) survey, 25% of the study sample of patients undergoing lipid management had TG concentrations ≥200 mg dl^{-1} [3]. A majority of these patients had not achieved their NCEP ATP III non-HDL-C goal, particularly among those with CHD or risk equivalents, in whom only 27% had a non-HDL-C level below 130 mg dl^{-1}.

6.1 CLINICAL FACTORS ASSOCIATED WITH ELEVATED TG AND NON-HDL-C LEVELS

Several clinical factors are associated with elevated TG and non-HDL-C concentrations including:

- overweight and obesity

- physical inactivity

- cigarette smoking

- excess alcohol intake

- high carbohydrate diets (>60% of energy)

- diseases (e.g. diabetes, nephritic syndrome, hypothyroidism) and

- medications (e.g. corticosteroids, estrogens, retinoids, beta-adrenergic blockers, protease inhibitors).

Several genetic conditions can also produce hypertriglyceridemia. For this reason, it is often prudent to screen first-degree relatives when a patient with very high TG levels is identified.

6.2 DISORDERS OF TG-RICH LIPOPROTEIN CLEARANCE

When conditions are present that impede the clearance of TG-rich lipoproteins in the circulation, the result can be levels of TGs high enough to increase the risk for pancreatitis. These include familial lipoprotein lipase deficiency (homo- or heterozygous) and apolipoprotein (Apo) CII deficiency. In the former, lipoprotein lipase, the primary enzyme involved in hydrolysis of TG molecules in circulating lipoproteins is deficient. In the latter case, there is a deficiency of Apo CII, which activates lipoprotein lipase, resulting in a functional deficit of lipoprotein lipase activity. These conditions often remain undiagnosed until some precipitating event, such as pregnancy or weight gain, causes the TG level to increase dramatically.

Other conditions that can impede clearance of TG-rich lipoproteins are dysbetalipoproteinemia and hepatic lipase deficiency. Dysbetalipoproteinemia results from a defective form of Apo E (Apo E2) that does not bind normally with hepatic receptors involved in the clearance of remnants of chylomicron and very-low-density lipoprotein (VLDL) particles. A physical finding that is sometimes present in these individuals is yellow-orange lines in the creases of the palms (striae palmaris), which result from cholesterol deposits.

In hepatic lipase deficiency, levels of small VLDL and intermediate-density lipoprotein (IDL) particles are elevated because the hepatic lipase enzyme is involved in the remodeling of these particles. However, because hepatic lipase also influences remodeling and catabolism of high-density lipoprotein (HDL) particles, the HDL-C level is also typically high when this hepatic lipase deficiency is present.

While clinicians should be aware of the aforementioned conditions, the vast majority of cases of hypertriglyceridemia have multifactorial causes and evaluation of the underlying genetics is only required in situations where the hypertriglyceridemia is severe or associated with sequelae such as pancreatitis. In such cases, referral to a lipid specialist is usually warranted.

6.3 INSULIN RESISTANCE AND HYPERTRIGLYCERIDEMIA

The most common causes of hypertriglyceridemia in the United States of America are being overweight and obesity and the insulin resistance that accompanies these conditions. Since insulin resistance is a central pathophysiologic determinant of the metabolic syndrome, many patients with elevated TGs ($\geq$150 mg dl^{-1}) will qualify for a metabolic syndrome diagnosis.

6.4 EXCESSIVE PRODUCTION OF VLDL: THE PRIMARY LIPID ABNORMALITY IN THE INSULIN-RESISTANT STATE

The primary metabolic abnormality associated with insulin-resistant states, including obesity and the metabolic syndrome, is overproduction of VLDL. Since newly secreted VLDL particles are TG-rich, the result is mild to moderate hypertriglyceridemia. If the overproduction of VLDL is accompanied by other defects, such as Apo CII deficiency, or a defect in the hepatic clearance of TG-rich lipoproteins, the result can be more severe hypertriglyceridemia.

Two features of the insulin-resistant state are centrally involved in the pathogenesis of VLDL overproduction: elevated circulating levels of free fatty acids (FFA) and hyperinsulinemia. It appears that both must be present to generate overproduction of VLDL. For example, in subjects with normal insulin sensitivity, a glucose infusion will increase the plasma insulin concentration, but also reduce levels of FFA and lower hepatic VLDL secretion [4]. In contrast, patients with poorly controlled type 1 diabetes have low insulin levels and high circulating concentrations of FFA, but do not have elevated VLDL secretion [4]. Among insulin-resistant individuals, particularly those with abdominal obesity, fasting and postprandial levels of circulating insulin are elevated, but this hyperinsulinemia does not suppress FFA release into the circulation to a normal degree, thus both insulin and FFA levels are elevated, resulting in VLDL overproduction.

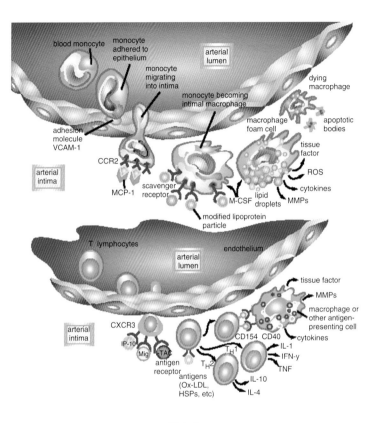

Plate 1

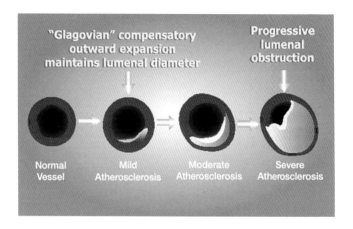

Plate 2

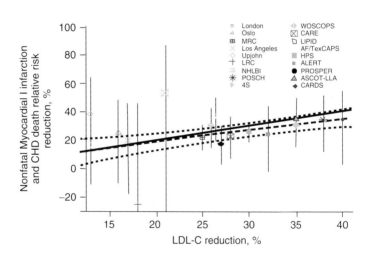

Plate 3

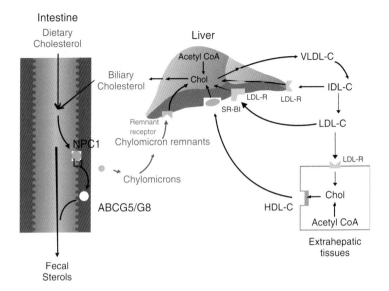

Intestine
Dietary Cholesterol

Liver

Acetyl CoA
Chol

Biliary Cholesterol

VLDL-C
IDL-C

LDL-R   LDL-R

Remnant receptor
Chylomicron remnants

SR-BI

LDL-C

NPC1
L1

Chylomicrons

ABCG5/G8

HDL-C

LDL-R

Chol

Acetyl CoA

Extrahepatic tissues

Fecal Sterols

Plate 4

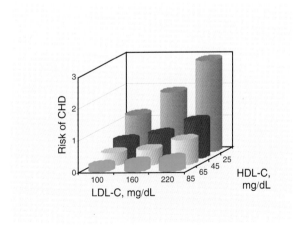

Risk of CHD

LDL-C, mg/dL

HDL-C, mg/dL

Plate 5

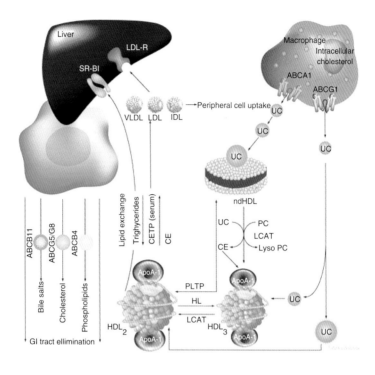

Plate 6

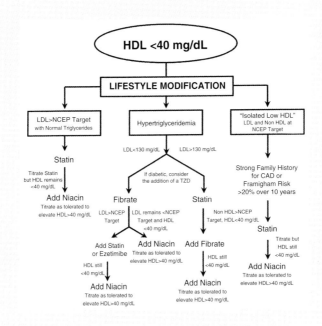

Plate 7

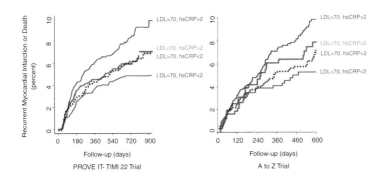

Plate 8

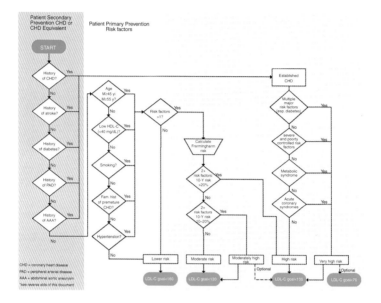

Plate 9

6.5 REASONS FOR ELEVATED FREE FATTY ACID LEVELS IN INSULIN-RESISTANT STATES

The release of FFA into the circulation is directly proportionate to the size of fat cells. Thus, being overweight and obesity are accompanied by greater release of FFA into the circulation. A chronically elevated FFA level is a cause of insulin resistance. This is illustrated by the observation that insulin resistance can be induced in normal subjects by the infusion of Intralipid (Pfizer, New York, NY) for several hours, which raises the FFA concentration, mimicking the obese state. The mechanisms that are responsible for the effects of a chronically elevated FFA level on insulin sensitivity are beyond the scope of this book, but the interested reader is referred to a recently published review on this topic [5].

6.6 BODY FAT DISTRIBUTION AND INSULIN RESISTANCE

FFA turnover in adipose tissues varies according to location. The abdominal visceral fat depots are the most metabolically active and contribute disproportionately to the circulating FFA level. For example, it has been estimated that an abdominally obese male with 20% of his body fat in the visceral stores will have a 50% contribution of these stores to the circulating FFA concentration [6]. Upper body subcutaneous fat is less metabolically active than abdominal visceral fat and lower body subcutaneous fat is least metabolically active. For this reason, an abdominally obese woman (apple shape) is likely to have greater lipid disturbances than a woman of similar body mass index (BMI) with a gynoid (pear shape) pattern of obesity, who carries most of her excess adiposity on the hips and thighs. Some ethnic groups (e.g. Asian Indians) tend to have a greater proportion of their body fat carried in the abdominal visceral depots, thus may display insulin resistance and other metabolic abnormalities at relatively low body weights.

6.7 INSULIN RESISTANCE IN THE NONOBESE PATIENT

It should be noted that an elevated circulating FFA concentration may be present in the absence of obesity [4]. In some individuals, the primary metabolic defect responsible for insulin resistance may be impaired "fat trapping." When TGs in lipoproteins are hydrolyzed, they enter cells (primarily adipose and muscle) through the action of acylation stimulating protein [7].

If this mechanism is impaired, the result is an abnormally large escape of FFA back into the circulation. Such people may have circulating FFA levels that are much higher than would be predicted by their degree of adiposity, and they may be thought of as being "metabolically obese" [7]. In addition, some medications, particularly antiretroviral drugs, may cause peripheral lipodystrophy with a resulting inability of subcutaneous adipose tissues to take up FFA released by lipoprotein lipase-catalyzed hydrolysis of TG, producing excess return of FFA liberated to the circulation and insulin resistance.

6.8 HYPERTRIGLYCERIDEMIA AND THE DEVELOPMENT OF ATHEROGENIC DYSLIPIDEMIA

Individuals with hypertriglyceridemia often have a triad of lipid disturbances that are termed *atherogenic dyslipidemia* by the NCEP ATP III [1]. The characteristic features of atherogenic dyslipidemia are:

1. elevated TGs;
2. depressed HDL-C;
3. a predominance of small, dense low-density lipoprotein (LDL) particles (LDL subclass pattern B).

An increase in the circulating TG concentration provides additional substrate for cholesteryl ester transfer protein (CETP), which catalyzes the exchange of TG from TG-rich lipoproteins to LDL and HDL particles in exchange for cholesteryl esters (Figure 6.1). The result is that the LDL and HDL particles become relatively TG rich and cholesterol poor. The TG in these particles can be hydrolyzed by hepatic lipase to form smaller, denser LDL and HDL particles.

Small, dense LDL particles are believed to have enhanced atherogenicity for several reasons [9, 10]. They have less affinity for the Apo B receptor, resulting in extended circulation in the plasma before hepatic clearance. Small, dense LDL particles also have greater interactivity with intra-arterial proteoglycans, which can lead to greater residence time within the arterial wall. Moreover, once in the arterial wall, they are more susceptible to oxidative modification. This can lead to unregulated uptake by macrophages, contributing to foam cell formation. However, this should not be interpreted to mean that larger, more buoyant LDL particles are benign. Data from several studies suggest that both large and small LDL particles are associated with increased CHD event risk and more severe atherosclerosis [11].

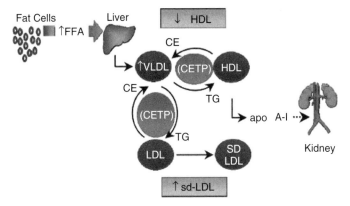

Figure 6.1 Metabolic pathways central to the development of the atherogenic dyslipidemia associated with insulin resistance and obesity: the lipid triad of hyper-triglyceridemia, depressed high-density lipoprotein cholesterol and small, dense low-density lipoprotein particles. FFA, free fatty acids; HDL, high-density lipoprotein; VLDL, very low-density lipoprotein; LDL, low-density lipoprotein; sd-LDL, small, dense low-density lipoproteins; CE, cholesteryl ester; CETP, cholesteryl ester transfer protein; TG, triglycerides; Apo, apolipoprotein. Adapted from Ginsberg, H.N. (2000) Insulin resistance and cardiovascular disease. *The Journal of Clinical Investigation*, **106**, 453–58, [8].

6.9 LIFESTYLE MANAGEMENT FOR THE METABOLIC SYNDROME AND ATHEROGENIC DYSLIPIDEMIA

A twofold approach is recommended for the management of the metabolic syndrome and atherogenic dyslipidemia [12]. The first is to reduce the under-lying lifestyle factors that contribute to the development of the insulin-resistant state, particularly obesity and physical inactivity. The second is to treat the individual lipid and nonlipid risk factors.

The NCEP ATP III has emphasized lifestyle changes as the first step in the management of the metabolic syndrome, insulin resistance, and the related risk factors, including atherogenic dyslipidemia. The two corner-stones of lifestyle changes for insulin-resistant patients are increased physical activity and loss of excess body fat. Both exercise and weight loss improve insulin sensitivity and all of the metabolic syndrome risk factors.

Cigarette smoking has also been shown to reduce insulin sensitivity and contribute to atherogenic dyslipidemia, adding to the myriad of rea-sons that smoking cessation should be encouraged. In addition, excessive alcohol intake will increase the TG concentration. Therefore, moderation (or cessation) of alcohol consumption should be encouraged if applicable [12].

In addition to the lifestyle changes outlined above, clinicians should be aware that some drug therapies can worsen the components of atherogenic dyslipidemia, and should thus be avoided if possible. These include oral estrogens (transdermal estrogens are a better alternative), retinoids (e.g. Accutane, Roche Pharmaceuticals, Basel, Switzerland), beta-adrenergic blockers, and thiazide diuretics [12].

6.10   DRUG THERAPIES

The primary target for lipid management is LDL-C. Once the LDL-C treatment goal has been achieved, additional strategies may be required if the non-HDL-C concentration remains above the treatment goal. There are two approaches to achieving non-HDL-C treatment goals in patients with high TG despite having achieved their LDL-C treatment goal. Often such patients will be taking a "standard" dose of a statin drug [2]. One approach is to further lower LDL-C by increasing the statin dose, adding a cholesterol absorption inhibitor, or by intensification of nondrug therapies [13, 14]. The other is to add an agent that primarily lowers VLDL-C and TG-rich remnant lipoproteins (a fibrate, niacin, or omega-3 fatty acids). At present, no clear evidence from clinical trials is available that would clearly favor one of these approaches.

6.11   INTENSIFICATION OF EFFORTS TO LOWER LDL-C AS A MEANS OF ACHIEVING THE NON-HDL-C GOAL

Statins are recommended as first-line therapy for patients with elevated LDL-C. However, statins also markedly reduce concentrations of both TG and TG-rich lipoproteins in hypertriglyceridemic subjects [15, 16]. The hypotriglyceridemic effects of statins have been widely underappreciated, largely because few studies of statin therapy had been undertaken in hypertriglyceridemic subjects until recently. TG lowering with statins is modest in normotriglyceridemic subjects, but much more pronounced in those with hypertriglyceridemia.

The use of statins is supported by a greater quantity of clinical trial data than any other class of lipid-altering agent. The results from large event trials have consistently shown that statin therapy reduces CHD morbidity and mortality. These effects are present at all levels of baseline lipids studied, as well as in groups that would be expected to be enriched with insulin-resistant individuals, such as subjects with diabetes mellitus, hypertriglyceridemia, and hypertension [17].

While statin therapy is very safe and well tolerated at lower doses, a large portion (75–85%) of the maximal effects on LDL-C and non-HDL-C are achieved at the usual starting doses. Each additional doubling of the statin dose is associated with further reductions of only 5–7%, while the risks of liver and muscle toxicity increase in proportion to the daily dosage. For this reason, it is not unreasonable to consider using a submaximal dose of statin therapy in combination with another agent, rather than using the maximal approved statin doses.

Additional agents that may be considered for further lowering of LDL-C include nondrug therapies (plant sterols/stanols and viscous fibers) or a cholesterol absorption inhibitor. Bile acid sequestrants also reduce LDL-C when added to statin therapy, but tend to modestly increase the plasma TG concentration, thus are not ideal for patients with hypertriglyceridemia. Plant sterols/stanols or viscous fibers can be expected to provide roughly 10% additional lowering of LDL-C and non-HDL-C when added to statin therapy [14, 18]. Coadministration of a cholesterol absorption inhibitor (e.g. 10-mg ezetemibe) will generally lower the LDL-C and non-HDL-C concentrations by a further 10–20% [19].

6.12 TARGETING TRIGLYCERIDE-RICH LIPOPROTEIN REDUCTION AS A MEANS OF ACHIEVING NON-HDL-C GOAL

Fibrates, niacin, and omega-3 fatty acids all effectively lower VLDL-C and other TG-rich lipoproteins. The effects of these agents are summarized below.

6.13 FIBRATES

Fibrates work by stimulating peroxisome proliferator activated receptor-α (PPAR-α). This results in enhanced lipoprotein lipase expression, reduced hepatic production of Apo CIII (which inhibits lipoprotein lipase), and enhanced hepatic fat oxidation. In addition, fibrates increase the production rates of Apo AI and Apo AII.

At the usual dosages, fibrates lower the TG concentration by 30–50% and increase HDL-C by 10–25%. The LDL-C response to fibrate therapy is dependent on both the baseline TG and LDL-C concentrations. In patients with very high TG concentrations (≥ 500 mg dl^{-1}), the LDL-C level may rise. In patients with less severe hypertriglyceridemia, particularly those with concomitantly elevated LDL-C, the LDL-C concentration may be neutral or decline by as much as 20%.

Clinical outcomes trials with fibrate therapy have been generally supportive of a protective effect regarding cardiovascular events [20, 21]. However, the results are not as robust as those observed with statins. In primary and secondary prevention trials with clofibrate, gemfibrozil, bezafibrate, and fenofibrate, the median relative risk reduction for the primary outcome variable was ∼20% (range 4–49%), with four of nine trials reaching statistical significance for the primary outcome variable [20, 21].

Results from subgroup analyses indicate that the most favorable effects on cardiovascular events have been observed in subjects with elevated TG concentrations at baseline [22, 23]. For example, the Bezafibrate Infarction Prevention Study had a nonsignificant relative risk reduction of 7.3% in the overall study sample, but a 39.5% relative risk reduction among the quarter of the study sample with a baseline TG concentration ≥ 200 mg dl^{-1} [22]. Despite the fact that fibrates are most often used in clinical practice to treat hypertriglyceridemia, none of the published event trials have specifically recruited hypertriglyceridemic subjects.

6.14 NIACIN

The dramatic effects of niacin on the blood lipid profile were noted more than a half-century ago, but the mechanisms responsible for these have been poorly understood until recently. The effects of niacin on lipid metabolism are due to its ability to suppress FFA release from adipose tissues as well as inhibition of hepatic diacylglycerol acyltransferase (DGAT) [24]. The latter is an enzyme involved with TG synthesis and VLDL production. The results of these changes are enhanced hepatic Apo B degradation and reduced VLDL production. Niacin also markedly increases the number of circulating HDL particles by selectively inhibiting the uptake of Apo AI by hepatocytes, thus reducing the catabolic rate of HDL. Extended release niacin at a dose of 2 g day^{-1} will reduce the plasma TG concentration by 20–50%, increase HDL-C by 15–35%, and lower LDL-C by 5–25%.

Although niacin improves all of the features of atherogenic dyslipidemia, two issues raise concerns about its clinical usefulness in such patients. The first is flushing, which is experienced to some degree by most patients. Its intensity is diminished, but not eliminated, by a prescription, extended release preparation (Niaspan®, Abbott Laboratories, Abbott Park, IL, USA). This side effect is bothersome to many patients, which may limit compliance. The second issue associated with niacin use is the development of insulin resistance. One might predict that the reduced FFA release from adipose tissues would lead to improved insulin sensitivity. However, the reverse appears to be true, although the mechanism(s) responsible for this effect are poorly understood [25]. The use of niacin can cause people with mild glucose intolerance to convert to frank diabetes by worsening the degree of insulin resistance and therefore increasing demand on the pancreatic beta cells [25, 26]. For this reason, niacin should be used with caution in patients with insulin resistance or glucose intolerance.

6.15   OMEGA-3 FATTY ACIDS

The long chain omega-3 polyunsaturated fatty acids eicosapentaenoic acid (EPA) and docosahexaenoic acid (DHA), found in high concentrations in the oils of cold water fish, have been known for years to have a hypotriglyceridemic effect when consumed in high doses ($1-4$ g day^{-1} of EPA + DHA). Recently, a prescription preparation of concentrated omega-3 acid ethyl esters (Lovaza®, GlaxoSmithKline, Middlesex, UK) has been made available. This formulation requires fewer capsules to achieve a therapeutic dose of omega-3 fatty acids. A dosage of 3.4 g EPA + DHA can be obtained from four 1-g capsules, which is the equivalent of the EPA + DHA content of $11-12$ g of fish oil.

Omega-3 fatty acids reduce VLDL production by inhibiting DGAT, and possibly through a mild stimulatory effect on PPAR-α, thus increasing hepatic fat oxidation [27, 28]. The result is reduced hepatic synthesis and secretion of VLDL, with no apparent effect on hepatic uptake of Apo B-containing particles [27, 28]. Omega-3 fatty acids therefore reduce circulating levels of TG and VLDL-C ($25-50\%$). They also generally produce a small rise in HDL-C ($3-10\%$). As with fibrates, omega-3 fatty acids sometimes lower LDL-C modestly ($5-10\%$), particularly among subjects with high baseline LDL-C. However, in patients with more severe hypertriglyceridemia, the LDL-C concentration may rise [29]. Nevertheless, the reduction in VLDL-C is typically larger than the increase in LDL-C, so the net result is a reduction in cholesterol carried by atherogenic lipoproteins (non-HDL-C).

6.16   MANAGEMENT OF DIABETIC DYSLIPIDEMIA

Diabetic dyslipidemia is essentially atherogenic dyslipidemia that occurs in a person with diabetes mellitus. The fundamental principles of its management do not differ from those for a patient with insulin resistance in the absence of diabetes. However, diabetic dyslipidemia may be affected by the degrees of glycemic control and relative insulin deficiency, which can increase the variability in lipid levels, particularly serum TG.

It should also be noted that some medications for glycemic control influence lipid concentrations, particularly the thiazolidinediones. A meta-analysis comparing the effects of the two available thiazolidinediones [30] found that, pioglitazone (Actos®, Takeda Pharmaceuticals, Lincolnshire, IL, USA) lowered the TG concentration (40 mg dl^{-1}) and elevated HDL-C (4.6 mg dl^{-1}). Its effects on total and LDL-C were neutral. In contrast, rosiglitazone (Avandia®, GlaxoSmithKline, Middlesex, UK) had no significant effect on TGs, but raised HDL-C (2.6 mg dl^{-1}), LDL-C (15 mg dl^{-1}) and total cholesterol (21 mg dl^{-1}).

CONTROVERSY

DO WE NEED A TRIGLYCERIDE TREATMENT TARGET TO INSURE A PREDOMINANCE OF LARGER, MORE BUOYANT LDL PARTICLES?

The NCEP ATP III has taken the position that lipoprotein cholesterol levels should be the main focus of lipid therapy. Therefore, they have established targets for apolipoprotein B-containing lipoprotein cholesterol levels (LDL-C and non-HDL-C). As discussed elsewhere in this chapter, the non-HDL-C treatment goal may be achieved in a hypertriglyceridemic patient by lowering LDL-C, lowering TG-rich lipoproteins (mainly VLDL) or a combination of the two strategies. Implicit in this recommendation is the idea that two patients with the same non-HDL-C and HDL-C levels will have similar CHD risk, regardless of whether the non-HDL-C goal is achieved through LDL-C lowering or lowering of TG-rich lipoproteins. Consider the following two patients (Table 1):

Table 1

Patient 1	Patient 2
Total C = 160 mg dl^{-1}	Total C = 160 mg dl^{-1}
HDL-C = 46 mg dl^{-1}	HDL-C = 46 mg dl^{-1}
Non-HDL-C = 114 mg dl^{-1}	Non-HDL-C = 114 mg dl^{-1}
LDL-C = 99 mg dl^{-1}	LDL-C = 70 mg dl^{-1}
Triglycerides = 75 mg dl^{-1}	Triglycerides = 220 mg dl^{-1}
LDL subclass pattern = A	LDL subclass pattern = B

Do these two patients have similar CHD risk, based on their lipid profiles? Currently available data do not provide a clear answer and this is an area of intense debate.

Both patients are within their NCEP ATP III treatment goals for LDL-C <100 mg dl^{-1} and non-HDL-C <130 mg dl^{-1}. Patient 2 has lower LDL-C, but also has higher triglycerides and a predominance of small, dense LDL particles (LDL subclass pattern B). The NCEP ATP III position suggests that their CHD event risks are similar. Proponents of the hypothesis that small, dense LDL particles are more atherogenic than larger, more buoyant particles might view patient 2 as being at higher risk than patient 1.

Figure 1 shows the relationship between the fasting triglyceride concentration and the relative risk for a CHD event among men in the Framingham Heart Study. The pattern suggests that most of the increase in risk associated with hypertriglyceridemia may occur when the triglyceride level rises above 100 mg dl^{-1}, increasing in a graded fashion until the level rises to 300 mg dl^{-1}, beyond which little additional risk is apparent. One possible explanation for this "S-shaped" relationship is the association of elevated triglycerides with the small, dense LDL (pattern B) phenotype.

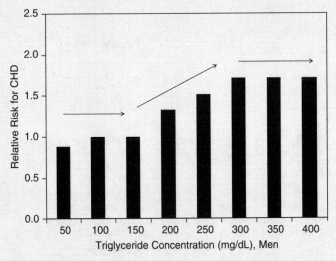

Figure 1 Relative risk of coronary heart disease (CHD) by serum triglyceride levels among men in the Framingham Heart Study (30-year follow-up). Adapted from Castelli, W.P. (1992) *The American Journal of Cardiology*, **70**, 3H-9H, [1].

Conversion between LDL subclass patterns appears to be a threshold phenomenon, with transition from pattern A to pattern B occurring when the fasting triglyceride level rises above a threshold level and the reverse occurring when the TG level falls below this level [2, 3]. The threshold varies between individuals, but is within the range of $100-250$ mg dl^{-1} for most of the population [2, 4]. This is illustrated in Figure 2, which shows the prevalence of pattern B as a function of the fasting triglyceride level. This relationship is also evident in clinical trials of triglyceride-lowering therapies. Figure 3 shows the prevalence of LDL subclass pattern B as a function of the on-treatment triglyceride level in a trial evaluating the lipid effects of adding prescription omega-3 treatment in men and women with persistent hypertriglyceridemia, despite statin therapy. Nearly all subjects had pattern B at baseline. Most subjects whose triglyceride level was lowered to below 150 mg dl^{-1} had pattern A while on treatment (64%), whereas most whose triglyceride level was 250 mg dl^{-1} or above showed pattern B (85%) during therapy, results that align well with the predictions based on the relationship shown in Figure 3.

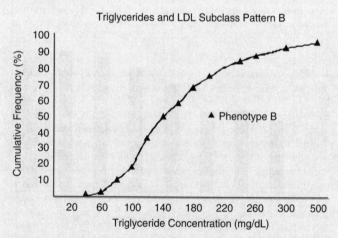

Figure 2   Association between fasting triglyceride level and the prevalence of low-density lipoprotein (LDL) subclass pattern B (a predominance of small, dense particles). Adapted from Austin, M.A. *et al.* (1990) *Circulation*, **82**, 495–506, [4].

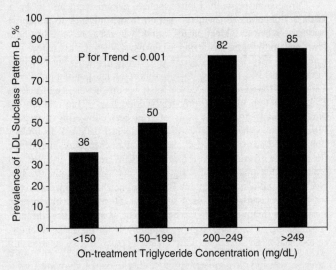

Figure 3 Prevalence of low-density lipoprotein (LDL) subclass pattern B by on-treatment triglyceride level among subjects taking simvastatin 40 mg d^{-1} plus prescription omega-3 acid ethyl esters 4 g d^{-1}. From Maki, K.C. *et al.* (2007) *The FASEB Journal*, (abstract 23.2), [3].

Thus, among those with markedly elevated triglyceride concentrations, even very large reductions in the triglyceride level induced by drug therapies will not generally produce an increase in LDL particle size unless the triglyceride level is reduced below the individual's threshold for conversion from pattern B to pattern A [2, 3]. Table 2 shows changes in lipid concentrations in response to fenofibrate therapy in subsets of subjects matched for the degree of triglyceride lowering, but differing with regard to the on-treatment TG concentration <200 or ≥200 mg dl^{-1}. Despite the same median percent reduction (and larger median absolute reduction) in triglycerides, subjects whose triglyceride level remained ≥200 mg dl^{-1} had no increase in median LDL particle size, whereas those whose triglycerides dropped below 200 mg dl^{-1} showed substantial increases in LDL particle diameter.

As reviewed by Packard [5], small, dense LDL particles bind less readily to hepatic receptors, prolonging their time in the circulation.

Table 2 Responses to fenofibrate therapy in hypertriglyceridemic subjects matched for percent change in triglyceride concentration, but differing in end-of-treatment triglyceride level (<200 and ≥ 200 mg dl^{-1}).

Variable	EOT triglycerides <200 mg dl^{-1}	EOT triglycerides ≥ 200 mg dl^{-1}	P-value
	Median change from baseline		
Triglycerides	−52%	−52%	0.927
LDL-C	4%	24%	0.229
Non-HDL-C	−18%	−15%	0.164
HDL-C	15%	19%	0.983
LDL particle size	0.79 nm	−0.06 nm	0.003

EOT, end-of-treatment; LDL-C, low-density lipoprotein cholesterol; non-HDL-C, non-high-density lipoprotein cholesterol; HDL-C, high-density lipoprotein cholesterol.

From Davidson, M.H. *et al.* (2006) *Clinical Cardiology*, **29**, 268–73, [2].

In contrast, these particles bind more readily to proteoglycans in the arterial wall and have greater susceptibility to oxidative modification, an important step in unregulated LDL uptake by macrophages during foam cell formation. However, despite the strong theoretical basis for the idea that small, dense LDL particles have enhanced atherogenicity, this has been difficult to demonstrate because the LDL subclass pattern is only one component of a larger group of metabolic characteristics including elevated triglycerides, low HDL-C, obesity, and insulin resistance [2, 4, 6, 7]. In a review of 70 studies evaluating the relationship of CHD risk with LDL particle size and number, small LDL particle size was found to be significantly associated with CHD risk in nearly all of the studies. However, in multivariate analyses, LDL size was rarely found to be a significant predictor of CHD risk, suggesting that other features associated with LDL particle size may account for part or all of its association with CHD risk [8].

In the Veterans Affairs High-Density Lipoprotein Intervention Trial (VA-HIT), both large and small LDL particle concentrations, but not LDL particle size, were significantly associated with CHD events once their correlation was taken into account [9]. Consistent with this finding, results from the Multi-Ethnic Study of Atherosclerosis (MESA) showed that both small and large LDL particles were associated with greater carotid intimal medial thickness (a surrogate for atherosclerosis) in models that adjusted for the inverse correlation between the two particle types (Table 3) [10].

Table 3 Associations of large and small low-density lipoprotein particle concentrations with carotid intimal-medial thickness after adjustment for low-density lipoprotein cholesterol, high-density lipoprotein cholesterol, and triglyceride concentrations in the Multi-Ethnic Study of Atherosclerosis.

Parameter	Difference (SE) in IMT (μm per SD)[a]	P value
Large LDL-P	30.3 (9.4)	0.001
Small LDL-P	34.8 (10.1)	0.001
LDL-C	11.8 (7.8)	0.130
HDL-C	−17.3 (5.7)	0.003
Triglycerides	−1.6 (5.1)	0.750

[a]Model also included terms for age, sex, race, hypertension, and smoking.
[b]HDL-C, high-density lipoprotein cholesterol; IMT, intimal-medial thickness; LDL-C, low-density lipoprotein cholesterol; LDL-P, low-density lipoprotein particle; SD, standard deviation; SE, standard error.
Adapted from Mora, S. *et al.* (2006) *Atherosclerosis*, **192**, 211S–17S, [10].

In addition, data from a variety of sources have supported the atherogenicity of remnants of triglyceride-rich particles such as intermediate density lipoproteins and chylomicron remnants [11]. Thus, the relative atherogenicity of various apolipoprotein B-containing particles is uncertain, leading one prominent authority in the field to declare [12]:

For the practicing clinician, however, the major argument for extending measurement of subclasses into the mass market is the hypothesis that one subclass is more atherogenic than another. Because evidence clearly indicates that all apolipoprotein B-containing particles are atherogenic, this reasoning is akin to the argument that an Uzi submachine gun is more deadly than an M16 or an AK47. Obviously all are potentially lethal, and although this assertion may interest gun aficionados, it matters little to law enforcement or to general public safety if the sole objective is disarmament!

While the authors believe that clinical trials are needed to test the hypothesis that lowering triglycerides to a target level might enhance CHD risk reduction by facilitating conversion to LDL subclass pattern A, we also feel that the data currently available are not sufficiently strong to advocate measurement of LDL particle size in clinical practice, or to justify the establishment of a triglyceride target. Therefore, until more data are available, we advocate focusing on efforts to achieve LDL-C (primary) and non-HDL-C (secondary) targets. Once these goals have been achieved, the clinician may opt to pursue further triglyceride reduction as a tertiary objective.

REFERENCES

[1] Castelli, W.P. (1992) Epidemiology of triglycerides: a view from Framingham. *The American Journal of Cardiology*, **70**, 3H–9H.
[2] Davidson, M.H., Bays, H.E., Stein, E. *et al*. (2006) Effects of fenofibrate on atherogenic dyslipidemia in hypertriglyceridemic subjects. *Clinical Cardiology*, **29**, 268–73.
[3] Maki, K.C., Davidson, M.H., Bays, H.E. *et al*. (2007) Effects of Omega-3-Acid Ethyl Esters on LDL Particle Size in Subjects with Hypertriglyceridemia Despite Statin Therapy. Proceedings of the Experimental Biology Meeting, Washington DC, Abstract # 231.2.
[4] Austin, M.A., King, M.C., Vranizan, K.M. and Krauss, R.M. (1990) Atherogenic lipoprotein phenotype: a proposed genetic marker for coronary heart disease risk. *Circulation*, **82**, 495–506.
[5] Packard, C.J. (2003) Triacylglycerol-rich lipoproteins and the generation of small, dense low-density lipoprotein. *Biochemical Society Transactions*, **31**, 1066–69.
[6] Maki, K.C., Davidson, M.H., Cyrowski, M.S. *et al*. (2000) Low-density lipoprotein subclass distribution pattern and adiposity-associated dyslipidemia in postmenopausal women. *Journal of the American College of Nutrition*, **19**, 23–30.
[7] Rizzo, M. and Berneis, K. (2007) Small, dense low-density-lipoproteins and the metabolic syndrome. *Diabetes Metabolism Research and Reviews*, **23**, 14–20.
[8] Cromwell, W.C. and Otvos, J.D. (2004) Low-density lipoprotein particle number and risk for cardiovascular disease. *Current Atherosclerosis Reports*, **6**, 381–87.
[9] Otvos, J.D., Collins, D., Freedman, D.S. *et al*. (2006) Low-density lipoprotein and high-density lipoprotein particle subclasses predict coronary events and are favorable changes by gemfibrozil therapy in the Veterans Affairs High-Density Lipoprotein Intervention Trial. *Circulation*, **113**, 1556–63.
[10] Mora, S., Szklo, M., Otvos, J.D., *et al*. (2006) LDL particle subclasses, LDL particle size, and carotid atherosclerosis in the Multi-Ethnic Study of Atherosclerosis (MESA). *Atherosclerosis*, **192**, 211S–17S.
[11] National Cholesterol Education Program. National Heart, Lung, and Blood Institute. National Institutes of Health. (2002) Third report of the National Cholesterol Education Program (NCEP) Expert Panel on Detection, Evaluation, and Treatment of High Blood Cholesterol in Adults

(Adult Treatment Panel III), Final Report. NIH Publication No. 02-5215. September 2002.
[12] Stein, E.A. (2006) Are measurements of LDL particles ready for prime time? *Clinical Chemistry*, **52**, 1643–44.

REFERENCES

[1] Expert Panel on Detection, Evaluation and Treatment of High Blood Cholesterol in Adults (2001) Executive summary of the third report of the National Cholesterol Education Program (NCEP) Expert Panel on Detection, Evaluation, and Treatment of High Blood Cholesterol in Adults (Adult Treatment Panel III). *The Journal of the American Medical Association*, **285**, 2486–97.

[2] Grundy, S.M., Cleeman, J.I., Bairey, C.N. *et al.* (2004) Implications of recent clinical trials for the National Cholesterol Education Program Adult Treatment Panel III guidelines. *Circulation*, **110**, 227–39.

[3] Davidson, M.H., Maki, K.C., Pearson, T.A. *et al.* (2005) Results of the National Cholesterol Education Program (NCEP) Evaluation Project Utilizing Novel E-Technology (NEPTUNE) II survey and implications for treatment under the recent NCEP Writing Group recommendations. *The American Journal of Cardiology*, **96**, 556–63.

[4] Reaven, G.M. (1997) Syndrome X: Past, present and future, *Clinical Research in Diabetes and Obesity, Volume II: Diabetes and Obesity*, Humana Press, Totowa, NJ, pp. 357–77.

[5] Boden, G. (2006) Fatty acid-induced inflammation and insulin resistance in skeletal muscle and liver. *Current Diabetes Reports*, **6**, 177–81.

[6] Bjorntorp, P. (1993) Visceral obesity: a "civilization syndrome". *Obesity Research*, **1**, 206–22.

[7] Sniderman, A.D., Cianflone, K., Arner, P. *et al.* (1998) The adipocyte, fatty acid trapping, and atherogenesis. *Arteriosclerosis, Thrombosis, and Vascular Biology*, **18**, 147–51.

[8] Ginsberg, H.N. (2000) Insulin resistance and cardiovascular disease. *The Journal of Clinical Investigation*, **106**, 453–58.

[9] Packard, C.J. (2003) Triacylglycerol-rich lipoproteins and the generation of small, dense low-density lipoprotein. *Biochemical Society Transactions*, **31** (Pt 5), 1066–69.

[10] Krauss, R.M. (1995) Dense low density lipoproteins and coronary artery disease. *The American Journal of Cardiology*, **75**, 53B–57B.

[11] Cromwell, W.C. and Otvos, J.D. (2007) Utilization of lipoprotein subfractions, in *Therapeutic Lipidology* (eds M.H. Davidson, P.P. Toth and K.C. Maki), Humana Press, Totowa, NJ.

[12] National Cholesterol Education Program (2002) Third Report of the National Cholesterol Education Program Expert Panel on Detection, Evaluation, and Treatment of High Blood Cholesterol in Adults, NIH Publication No. 02-5215.

[13] Grundy, S.M. (2002) Low-density lipoprotein, non-high-density lipoprotein, and apolipoprotein B as targets of lipid-lowering therapy. *Circulation*, **106**, 2526–29.

[14] Maki, K.C., Galant, R. and Davidson, M.H. (2005) Non-high-density lipoprotein cholesterol: the forgotten therapeutic target. *The American Journal of Cardiology*, **96** (Suppl 9A), 59K–64K.

[15] Isaacsohn, J., Hunninghake, D., Schrott, H. *et al.* (2003) Effects of simvastatin, an HMG-CoA reductase inhibitor, in patients with hypertriglyceridemia. *Clinical Cardiology*, **26**, 18–24.

[16] Watts, G.F., Barrett, P.H., Ji, J. *et al.* (2003) Differential regulation of lipoprotein kinetics by atorvastatin and fenofibrate in subjects with the metabolic syndrome. *Diabetes*, **52**, 803–11.

[17] Cholesterol Treatment Trialists' Collaboration (2005) Efficacy and safety of cholesterol-lowering treatment: prospective meta-analysis of data from 90,056 participants in 14 randomised trials of statins. *Lancet*, **366**, 1267–78.

[18] Katan, M.B., Grundy, S.M., Jones, P. *et al.* (2003) Efficacy and safety of plant stanols and sterols in the management of blood cholesterol levels. *Mayo Clinic Proceedings*, **78**, 965–78.

[19] Davidson, M.H., McGarry, T., Bettis, R. *et al.* (2002) Ezetimibe coadministered with simvastatin in patients with primary hypercholesterolemia. *Journal of the American College of Cardiology*, **40**, 2125i–34i.

[20] Maki, K.C. (2004) Fibrates for treatment of the metabolic syndrome. *Current Atherosclerosis Reports*, **6**, 45–51.

[21] FIELD Investigators (2005) Effects of long-term fenofibrate therapy on cardiovascular events in 9795 people with type 2 diabetes mellitus (the FIELD Study): randomised controlled trial. *Lancet*, **366**, 1849–61.

[22] BIP Study Group (2000) Secondary prevention by raising HDL cholesterol and reducing triglycerides in patients with coronary artery disease: the Bezafibrate Infarction Prevention (BIP) Study. *Circulation*, **102**, 21–27.

[23] Robins, S.J., Collins, D., Wittes, J.T. *et al.* (2001) Relation of gemfibrozil treatment and lipid levels with major coronary events VA-HIT: a randomized controlled trial. *The Journal of the American Medical Association*, **285**, 1585–91.

[24] Ganji, S.H., Kamanna, V.S. and Kashyap, M.L. (2003) Niacin and cholesterol: role in cardiovascular disease (review). *The Journal of Nutritional Biochemistry*, **14**, 298–305.

[25] Ginsberg, H.N. (2006) Niacin in the metabolic syndrome: more risk than benefit? *Nature Clinical Practice Endocrinology and Metabolism*, **2**, 300–1.

[26] Kahn, S.E., Prigeon, R.L., Schwartz, R.S. *et al.* (2001) Obesity, body fat distribution, insulin sensitivity and islet beta-cell function as explanations for metabolic diversity. *The Journal of Nutrition*, **131**, 354S–60S.

[27] Chan, D.C., Watts, G.F., Barrett, P.H. *et al.* (2002) Regulatory effects of HMG CoA reductase inhibitor and fish oils on apolipoprotein B-100 kinetics in insulin-resistant obese male subjects with dyslipidemia. *Diabetes*, **51**, 2377–86.

[28] Chan, D.C., Watts, G.F., Mori, T.A. *et al.* (2003) Randomized controlled trial of the effect of n-3 fatty acid supplementation on the metabolism of apolipoprotein B-100 and chylomicron remnants in men with visceral obesity. *The American Journal of Clinical Nutrition*, **77**, 300–7.

[29] Bays, H.E. (2006) Clinical overview of Omacor: a concentrated formulation of omega-3 polyunsaturated fatty acids. *The American Journal of Cardiology*, **98** (4A), 71i–76i.

[30] Chiquette, E., Ramirez, G. and DeFronzo, R. (2004) A meta-analysis comparing the effect of thiazolidinediones on cardiovascular risk factors. *Archives of Internal Medicine*, **164**, 2097–104.

7 Management of Depressed High-density Lipoprotein Cholesterol

Key Points

- *Low serum levels of high-density lipoprotein cholesterol (HDL-C) are an independent risk factor for cardiovascular disease (CVD) in both men and women.*

- *The HDLs can potentiate a number of antiatherosclerotic effects, including reverse cholesterol transport (RCT) and a variety of antioxidative, antithrombotic, and anti-inflammatory effects along vessel walls.*

- *HDL-C can be increased in patients with dyslipidemia using statins, fibrates, niacin, thiazolidinediones, and, in peri- and postmenopausal women in the short-term, estrogen.*

- *Considerable investment is being made to develop newer pharmacologic agents that will impact HDL metabolism in an effort to further reduce risk for cardiovascular events in both the primary and secondary prevention settings.*

Of the various lipoproteins targeted for therapeutic management, none of them are as challenging or problematic to treat as the high-density lipoproteins or HDLs. The metabolism of HDLs is complex and these lipoproteins appear to exert a variety of antiatherogenic effects. There are numerous enzymes, cell surface receptors, and genetic and metabolic backgrounds that impact on serum levels of HDL. Given the large number of polymorphisms regulating HDL levels, specific lifestyle modifications and pharmacologic interventions can have quite variable effects on HDL levels following therapeutic manipulation. The management of low HDL is recognized as being

Practical Lipid Management: Concepts and Controversies   Peter P. Toth and Kevin C. Maki
© 2008 John Wiley & Sons, Ltd

clinically important by both American and European guidelines for CVD risk reduction. Simply targeting low-density lipoprotein cholesterol (LDL-C) reduction leaves the majority of patients in clinical trials at risk for acute CVD related events, such as myocardial infarction (MI) stroke, and sudden death. This chapter will review the epidemiology of HDL and its relationship to risk for developing atherosclerotic disease, the complex metabolism of HDL and its broad-ranging antiatherogenic effects, and the impact of lifestyle modification and drug therapy on serum levels of this lipoprotein.

7.1 THE RELATIONSHIP BETWEEN HDL AND RISK FOR CVD

The correlation between low HDL and increased risk for CVD is not a new concept. This relationship was first reported by Barr and coworkers in 1951 [1] and was confirmed less than 10 years later years later in an Israeli cohort [2]. Since the 1960s, epidemiologic studies performed throughout the world have substantiated this finding and have shown that low serum levels of HDL-C are an independent risk factor for CAD, stroke, peripheral arterial disease (PAD), premature atherosclerotic disease of the left main coronary artery, in-stent restenosis, and sudden death [3–7]. Low HDL-C is also associated with more rapid rates of atheromatous plaque progression compared with patients with normal levels of this lipoprotein. In contrast, elevated levels of HDL-C appear to protect both men and women from developing atherosclerotic disease.

The Framingham Study demonstrated that as HDL-C decreases, risk for CAD-related events increases at any level of LDL-C or total cholesterol [8]. The Framingham workers also showed that for every 20 mg dl^{-1} rise in HDL-C, risk for CAD was reduced by 50%. Moreover, at any serum level of LDL-C, as HDL-C progressively decreased, risk for coronary heart disease (CHD)-related events increased [9]. (Figure 7.1) The Cooperative Lipoprotein Phenotyping Study (CLPS) evaluated populations in five American locales, which included Albany, New York; Evans County, Georgia; Framingham, Massachusetts; Honolulu, Hawaii; and San Francisco, California. CLPS showed that as HDL decreases, risk for CAD increases independent of serum triglycerides and LDL-C [10]. Importantly, among men, the Physicians' Health Study [11] found that a low HDL-C increases risk for CAD even if total cholesterol is low, while the Tromso Heart Study showed that low HDL-C imparts a risk for CAD that is three times higher than if LDL-C is high [12]. Among European and Nordic populations, the Prospective Cardiovascular Munster Study, Prospective Epidemiological Study of

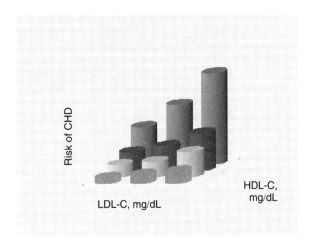

Figure 7.1 Risk for coronary heart disease (CHD) as a function of low-density lipoprotein cholesterol (LDL-C) and high-density lipoprotein cholesterol (HDL-C) in the Framingham Study. At any serum level of LDL-C, as HDL-C decreases, risk for CHD increases. The lowest risk for CHD appears to occur in study subjects with the lowest LDL-C and the highest HDL-C. Reproduced with permission from Castelli, W.P. (1988) *The Canadian Journal of Cardiology*, **4** (Suppl A), 5A–10A, [9]. A full-color version of this figure appears in the color plate section of this book.

Myocardial Infarction, and the Apolipoprotein-Related Mortality Risk Study all found that as serum HDL-C decreased, risk for acute cardiovascular events increased [13–15]. Among the elderly aged >75 years evaluated in the Northern Manhattan Stroke Study, HDL-C was inversely associated with risk for stroke, with a dose–response relationship [16]. In the Cardiovascular Health Study, elevated HDL-C protected men aged ≥65 years against MI and ischemic stroke in a dose–response manner [17].

A number of studies have quantified the relationship between serum HDL-C and CHD risk reduction. Among Japanese men residing in Osaka, for every 1 mg dl^{-1} rise in HDL-C, risk for CAD and MI decreases by 5.7 and 6.4%, respectively [18]. An aggregate analysis of the Framingham Study, the Multiple Risk Factor Intervention Trial, the Lipid research Clinics Primary Prevention Trial, and the Lipid Research Clinics Prevalence Mortality Follow-up Study demonstrated that for every 1 mg dl^{-1} rise in HDL-C, risk for CAD decreased by 2 and 3% for men and women, respectively [19]. In the Framingham Offspring Study, a 1 mg dl^{-1} elevation in

HDL was associated with a 2% reduction in risk for CHD [20]. Among women in the Nurses' Health Study, a 17% elevation in HDL-C correlated with a decrease in CHD risk of 40% [21]. In patients who sustain a non-Q wave MI and undergo drug-eluting stent placement, HDL-C <40 mg dl^{-1} compared with HDL-C ≥ 40 mg dl^{-1} portends a 3.3-fold higher risk of mortality after one year of follow-up [22]. In addition, this study also showed that in these patients, for every 1 mg dl^{-1} rise in serum HDL-C, risk for target lesion revascularization (repeat revascularization by percutaneous or surgical means within the stent or in the 5-mm distal or proximal segments adjacent to the stent) and major cardiac events was reduced by 4%. Increasing serum levels of HDL-C with statins is associated with reductions in coronary artery atheromatous plaque volume, independent of changes in LDL-C [23, 24].

7.2   PREVALENCE OF LOW HDL-C

Low serum levels of HDL-C are highly prevalent among patients with the metabolic syndrome, diabetes mellitus, as well as patients with atherosclerotic disease. The National Cholesterol Education Program (NCEP) defines a low HDL-C as <40 mg dl^{-1} and considers low HDL-C a categorical risk factor for CHD and its sequelae [25]. Among women, the American Heart Association has defined low HDL-C as <50 mg dl^{-1} since women tend to have an HDL-C that is on average 10 mg dl^{-1} higher compared to age matched men [26]. Patients who are diabetic or who have metabolic syndrome tend to have low serum levels of HDL-C because they are insulin resistant. As will be detailed below, insulin resistance can impair HDL biosynthesis and augment its catabolism, resulting in low levels of this lipoprotein. Approximately 25% of the population in the USA has the metabolic syndrome [27]. The incidence of the metabolic syndrome is growing rapidly worldwide, including Europe, Asia, and South America. In the USA, 39% of men and 15% of women have HDL-C <40 mg dl^{-1} [28]. In one analysis of patients with CAD or a CHD risk equivalent, 66% of patients had HDL-C <40 mg dl^{-1}, even if they were being treated with a statin and their LDL-C was treated to target levels [29]. Among Europeans diagnosed with dyslipidemia, the frequency of HDL levels <40 mg dl^{-1} in men and <50 mg dl^{-1} in women is 40 and 33%, respectively [30]. Among men with CAD and who receive their medical care through the Veterans Administration system, HDL <40 mg dl^{-1} occurs with a frequency of 64% [31]. In another series of patients discharged from an academic medical center following an acute coronary syndrome, coronary revascularization procedure, or an ischemic cerebrovascular accident, the prevalence of HDL-C <40 mg dl^{-1} was 69% [32]. The prevalence of low HDL-C is threefold higher among patients with premature CAD compared with healthy controls [33].

7.3   GOALS FOR HDL TREATMENT

Setting a goal for serum HDLs is a controversial issue. The NCEP has not defined a target for therapy for two primary reasons. First, there is no prospective, randomized clinical trial that has been able to define a target level in serum for this class of lipoproteins. One important feature of all forms of lifestyle modification and currently available pharmaco-logic interventions is that each of these therapeutic approaches impact on all components of the lipid profile, not just HDL-C. Getting an unequivo-cal answer to the question of how a therapy specifically impacts HDL-C and how a given change in HDL-C affects risk becomes challenging. Sec-ond, currently available medications do not impact HDL production and metabolism in a manner that is uniform enough to predict an individual patient's response either in the near- or long-term. Some patients may expe-rience a very brisk response to therapy and experience large elevations in HDL; others may only experience small elevations (2–5%) in response to therapy with polypharmacy and comprehensive lifestyle modification. When HDL-C is low, NCEP clearly recommends that therapeutic effort be made to raise HDL-C with therapeutic lifestyle change (TLC) (weight loss, aero-bic exercise, TLC diet, smoking cessation) and pharmacologic intervention as dictated by the specific features of a patient's lipid profile (discussed in greater detail below).

Other guideline writing groups have taken a more proactive and aggres-sive approach (Table 7.1). Among diabetic patients, the American Diabetes Association recommends that HDL-C be increased to >40 mg dl^{-1} and in women to >50 mg dl^{-1} [34]. The Expert Group on HDL Cholesterol [35] and the European Consensus Panel on HDL-C [36] recommend that HDL-C be increased to ≥ 40 mg dl^{-1} in patients with CAD, metabolic syndrome, diabetes mellitus, or a 10 years Framingham risk $\geq 20\%$.

Low HDL-C impacts on Framingham risk scores. For patients with HDL-C <40 mg dl^{-1}, two points are added to the 10 years Framing-ham risk score. If HDL-C exceeds 60 mg dl^{-1}, one point is subtracted from the Framingham risk score. An important point is that no matter how high HDL-C is, once it is >60 mg dl^{-1}, only one point can be subtracted from the total. Consequently, if a patient presents with an HDL-C of 80 or 90 mg dl^{-1}, can one assume that they will be protected against the develop-ment of atherosclerosis? *No*. In patients with two or more risk factors and

Table 7.1 Guideline definitions for low high-density lipoprotein cholesterol (HDL-C) and targets for therapy.

Guideline sponsor	Definition for low HDL-C
National Cholesterol Education Program	<40 mg dl^{-1} (all patients)[a]
American Heart Association	<50 mg dl^{-1} (women)

Guideline sponsor	HDL-C target for therapy
National Cholesterol Education Program	None
European Consensus Panel on HDL-C	≥ 40 mg dl^{-1} [b]
Expert Group on HDL-C	≥ 40 mg dl^{-1} [b]
American Diabetes Association	>40 mg dl^{-1} in men
	>50 mg dl^{-1} in women

[a]When diagnosing metabolic syndrome, NCEP defines low HDL-C as <40 mg dl^{-1} in men and <50 mg dl^{-1} in women.
[b]For patients with CAD and those at high risk for CAD (metabolic syndrome, diabetes mellitus, 10-year Framingham risk $>20\%$).

Taken from: Mosca, L. *et al.* (2004) *Arteriosclerosis, Thrombosis, and Vascular Biology*, **24**, e29–e50, [26]. Haffner, S.M. and American Diabetes Association (2004) *Diabetes Care*, **27**, S68–S71, [34]. Sacks, F.M. (2002) *The American Journal of Cardiology*, **90**, 139–43, [35]. Chapman, M.J. *et al.* (2004) *Current Medical Research and Opinion*, **20**, 1253–68, [36]. National Cholesterol Education Program (2002) Final Report, NIH Publication No. 02-5215, [37].

no CHD risk equivalents, the 10 years Framingham risk score should be calculated. One cannot assume that an elevated HDL-C will protect patients from atherosclerotic disease irrespective of the composition of their global risk factor burden.

7.4 ANTIATHEROGENIC EFFECTS OF HDL

Cholesterol is an important modulator of cell membrane fluidity and is a precursor to steroid hormones and bile salts. Cholesterol can be catabolized to bile salts by hepatocytes. Peripheral somatic cells such as those found in arterial vessel walls cannot clear excess amounts of cholesterol by breaking it down into smaller byproducts. As cholesterol accumulates in macrophages to form foam cells, internalized lipid droplets will expand continuously until the cell dies unless it is stimulated to externalize excess cholesterol. HDL particles drive RCT, the process by which HDL promotes the mobilization and externalization of excess cholesterol and delivers it back to the liver for disposal as either bile salts or biliary cholesterol (Figure 7.2). It is believed that RCT is among the most important antiatherogenic effects that HDL mediates (see [38] and references therein). Low serum levels of HDL may represent a state of reduced or inadequate capacity for RCT, leading to an excess accumulation of cholesterol in the subendothelial space of blood vessels [39, 40].

Apoprotein A-I (Apo A-I) is secreted from both the jejunum and liver. Free or non-lipidated Apo A-I can bind to phospholipids and form a hockey puck-like structure known as *nascent discoidal high-density lipoprotein* (ndHDL) (Figure 7.2). Both Apo A-I and ndHDL can bind to the surface of macrophages via the receptor ABCA1, or ATP binding membrane cassette transport protein A1. When ABCA1 is bound by these molecular species, it transports cholesterol from the cytosol into the extracellular space [42]. Externalized cholesterol is then esterified with a fatty acid to form cholesteryl esters by the enzyme lecithin cholesteryl acyltransferase (LCAT). Because cholesteryl esters are hydrophobic or poorly soluble in water, they become partitioned into the core of ndHDL. As more and more cholesteryl ester and phospholipids are incorporated into the particle, the ndHDL speciates and becomes progressively larger and more spherical, forming HDL_3 and HDL_2. Mutations that reduce the functionality of Apo A-I are associated with hypoalphalipoproteinemia and increased risk for CHD, while gain of function mutations in Apo A-I are associated with hyperalphalipoproteinemia and reduced risk for CHD. Mutations in ABCA1 that reduce its capacity to bind Apo A-I or translocate intracellular cholesterol result in hypoalphalipoproteinemia and increased risk for CHD [43–45]. Apo A-I and ndHDL that cannot be lipidated properly, are catabolized and cleared from the circulation.

HDL particles formed in this process can undergo a number of fates. HDL can transport cholesteryl esters to steroidogenic organs and facilitate steroid hormone biosynthesis. HDLs can interact with cholesteryl ester transfer protein, an enzyme that exchanges cholesteryl ester in HDL for triglycerides in Apo B-100-containing lipoproteins, such as very low-density lipoprotein (VLDL) and LDL. The cholesteryl esters transferred into these lipoproteins can be delivered to the liver via the LDL receptor and the LDL receptor-related protein (Figure 7.2). This is known as *indirect RCT*.

Direct RCT involves the binding of HDL to other receptors on the hepatocyte surface. Two of these have been characterized. The first is scavenger receptor B-I (SR-BI), a receptor that mediates selective cholesteryl ester uptake. HDL binds to SR-BI via its Apo A-I moiety [46]. After docking, cholesteryl esters are extracted, taken up into the hepatocyte, and the delipidated HDL particle is extruded back into the circulation to begin another round of RCT. The second involves a protein (the β-chain of the F_1 subunit of F_1F_0 ATP synthetase) that modulates holoparticle endocytosis of HDL [47]. The entire HDL particle is taken up by the hepatocyte and is catabolized. The cholesterol delivered back to the liver by HDL can undergo a variety of fates: (i) it can be repackaged into VLDL and secreted back

into the circulation; (ii) it can be catabolized to bile salts by the enzyme
7α-hydroxylase; and (iii) it can be secreted into bile and the gastrointestinal
tract unmodified. The process of RCT has been validated in both humans
and rodents [48, 49].

The HDLs are unique among the lipoproteins because rather than driving the net deposition of cholesterol into vessels walls, they promote its
extraction and delivery to the liver for catabolism and disposal. The HDLs
are also unusual because they participate in a variety of other reactions
believed to be antiatherogenic (summarized in Table 7.2). HDL increases
endothelial cell nitric oxide production, inhibits adhesion molecule expression, stimulates endothelial cell proliferation in areas of arterial injury, and
inhibits endothelial cell apoptosis (programmed cell death) [50–53]. These
changes are associated with increased vasodilatation, reduced inflammatory
tone, and integrity of the endothelial cell layer. Oxidized LDL is the main
substrate for foam cell formation. LDL is oxidized by a number of enzymes,
such as myeloperoxidase and 5′-lipoxygenase. HDL is able to reduce oxidized LDL. HDL is a carrier of paraoxonase, glutathione peroxidase, and
platelet activating factor acetylhydrolase [54, 55]. These three enzymes

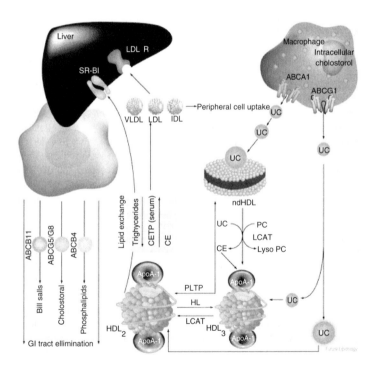

reduce oxidatively modified components of LDL. HDL also exerts a variety of antiplatelet and antithrombotic effects. HDL stimulates endothelial cell prostacyclin production, which is both vasodilatory and antithrombotic [56]. Hdls decrease platelet thromboxane A2 production and platelet aggregability, and potentiate urokinase mediated fibrinolysis and the ability of proteins C and S to inactivate coagulation factor Va [57–59].

Given the capacity of HDL to drive RCT and mediate a large number of antiatherogenic effects, the ability of HDL to reduce rates of atheromatous plaque progression and even induce its regression has been tested in a variety of animal models. Intravenously infusing Apo A-I into rabbits fed an atherogenic diet decreases atherosclerotic disease when compared with untreated controls [60]. Mice transfected with human Apo A-I undergo atheromatous plaque regression [61]. The intravenous infusion of HDL into rabbits without established atherosclerotic disease blocks its development

---

Figure 7.2   Pathways for reverse cholesterol transport. Macrophages resident in the intima of arterial walls develop into foam cells as they take up ever greater amounts cholesterol from modified LDL particles. Unlike hepatocytes, macrophages cannot metabolize cholesterol into excretory by-products. In order to maintain cholesterol homeostasis, macrophages express membrane-bound sterol transporter proteins that pump excess cholesterol into the extracellular space. Free Apo A-I or the ApoA-I in nascent discoidal HDL (ndHDL) binds to ABCA1 and induces sterol mobilization from intracellular lipid pools. Cholesterol and phospholipids are pumped out of the cell and bind to free apo A-I and ndHDL. Unesterified cholesterol (UC) esterified by LCAT on the surface of HDL particles using phosphatidylcholine as a fatty acid donor. The esterified cholesterol moves into the HDL particle's hydrophobic core along a concentration gradient. As more and more cholesteryl ester enters the HDL particle, it becomes spherical, resulting in the formation HDL_3 and then the larger HDL_2. These spherical HDL particles can stimulate additional cholesterol externalization through the translocator ABCG1. Reverse cholesterol transport (RCT) has evolved two distinct pathways: direct and indirect. During direct RCT, HDL binds to SR-BI on the hepatocyte surface. The HDL particle is selectively delipidated (i.e. its cholesteryl esters are removed). Once delipidation is complete, rather than catabolizing the particle into its constituent apoproteins and phospholipids, the HDL particle is released so as to initiate another cycle of RCT. Indirect RCT depends on lipid exchange catalyzed by CETP. During this reaction, the cholesteryl esters in HDL are exchanged for triglycerides carried in apoB100-containing lipoproteins such as VLDL, IDL, and LDL. The cholesteryl ester is carried back to the liver for systemic clearance by the LDL receptor (low-density lipoprotein receptor (LDL-R)). Cholesterol delivered back to the liver can either be excreted in bile as free cholesterol or converted into bile salts via 7-α-hydroxylase. Alternatively, the cholesterol can be repackaged into VLDL for hepatic secretion into the circulation. PLTP, phospholipid transfer protein; HL, hepatic lipase. Reproduced with permission from: Toth, P.P. (2007) *Future Lipidology*, **2**, 277–84, [41]. A full-color version of this figure appears in the color plate section of this book.

Table 7.2 Antiatherogenic functions of high-density lipoproteins.

Reverse cholesterol transport
Apoprotein donor to other lipoproteins
Inhibits matrix metalloproteinase production (can lead to lead plaque stabilization)
Stimulates angiogenesis

Antioxidative effects

1. Increase nitric oxide production and potentiate vasodilatation and myocardial perfusion
2. Suppress Vascular Cell Adhesion Molecule 1 (VCAM-1) and Intercellular Adhesion Molecule 1 (ICAM-1) expression
3. Promote endothelial progenitor cell recruitment and engraftment
4. Stimulate endothelial cell proliferation and migration
5. Inhibit apoptosis by blocking activation of caspases 3 and 9

Antioxidative effects

1. There are two redox-active methionine (amino acid sequence positions 112 and 148) residues in apo AI that reduce oxidized phospholipids, lipid peroxides and hydroperoxides, and oxidized cholesterol esters, in LDL via the activity of three antioxidative enzymes:

   i. Paraoxonase
   ii. Platelet activating factor acetylhydrolase
   iii. Glutathione peroxidase

Antithrombotic effects

Stimulates

1. Fibrinolysis
2. The ability of proteins C and S to inactivate coagulation factor Va
3. Prostacyclin production by activating cyclooxygenase-2

Inhibits

1. Thrombin-mediated platelet aggregation
2. Platelet activation
3. Platelet thromboxane A2 production
4. Tissue factor production

and stimulates plaque regression in animals with atherosclerosis [62]. The infusion of reconstituted native human Apo A-I into patients with CAD is associated with modest atheromatous plaque regression after only five once weekly injections [63].

7.5 HDL AND INSULIN RESISTANCE

Insulin resistance impacts on HDL metabolism significantly. Apo A-I is carried by chylomicron and VLDL particles. In the setting of insulin resistance, the activity of lipoprotein lipase is decreased. Lipoprotein lipase hydrolyzes the triglycerides in chylomicrons and VLDL, which results in the dissociation of Apo A-I and phospholipids from the surface of these particles. Through this release of "surface coat mass," dissociated Apo A-I and phospholipids can be used to assimilate HDL in serum. When lipoprotein lipase is inhibited, less surface coat mass is released and there is excess triglyceride available in serum. Cholesterol ester transfer protein (CETP) catalyzes the exchange of triglycerides for cholesteryl esters from VLDL to HDL and LDL. As the HDL and LDL become progressively more enriched with triglyceride, these lipoproteins become better substrates for catabolism by hepatic lipase (HL) and endothelial lipase [64, 65]. The LDL becomes smaller, denser, and more atherogenic. Similarly, the HDL becomes smaller, but also more unstable. As lipolysis continues, Apo A-I dissociates and the HDL particle is catabolized. When free Apo A-I is not lipidated, it can be bound by cubulin or megalin in the glomerular ultrafiltrate and eliminated from the body. HDL levels may also decrease in patients with insulin resistance because of decreased hepatic Apo A-I biosynthesis. Insulin resistance is a manifestation of increased visceral, not subcutaneous, adiposity, defined as increased adipose tissue mass in omental, perinephric, peritoneal, and perimesenteric depots. Weight loss and increased physical activity reduce and can even resolve insulin resistance.

7.6 EFFECTS OF LIFESTYLE MODIFICATION ON SERUM HDL

WEIGHT AND WEIGHT LOSS

In patients presenting with low serum levels of HDL-C, the NCEP guidelines recommend counseling about lifestyle modification. A variety of TLCs can favorably impact serum HDL-C. HDL-C decreases as a function of rising weight or body mass index and, as a general rule of thumb, for every 1 kg m^{-2} rise in fat mass, HDL-C decreases by 1 mg dl^{-1} [66, 67]. The opposite is also true: weight loss results in an increase in HDL-C [67]. During the acute phase of weight loss, HDL-C can decrease; however, once the patient's weight and diet stabilize, HDL-C will typically be higher than at baseline. Increased ingestion of *trans* fat and carbohydrate or decreased saturated fat intake lowers HDL-C [68–71]. A Mediterranean diet characterized by increased intake of legumes, olive oil, fruits, and vegetables has been shown to decrease insulin resistance and increase HDL-C [72].

EXERCISE

Increased exercise is always a key feature of any lifestyle modification plan, and regular exercise is associated with reduced risk for CVD. Both men and women tend to experience increasing weight with aging, some of which is due to decreased exercise frequency and intensity. There is a positive dose–response relationship between exercise duration and serum HDL-C [73, 74]. Importantly, exercise blunts the reduction in serum HDL-C when patients lose weight with low-fat diets [75]. Patients with hypertriglyceridemia at baseline tend to experience more robust elevations in HDL-C when they begin to exercise compared with their normotriglyceridemic counterparts [76].

CIGARETTE SMOKING

Cigarette smoking decreases serum HDL-C in a dose–response manner [77]. (Figure 7.3) Evidence suggests that cigarette smoking adversely impacts HDL metabolism by: (i) exacerbating insulin resistance [78] and (ii) decreasing the formation and maturation of HDL by inhibiting LCAT [79]. Smoking cessation can increase HDL-C by up to 20%, an elevation that is on par with the most efficacious pharmacologic interventions we currently have available [80]. Among smokers, smoking cessation should always be a part of any lifestyle modification program designed to raise HDL-C.

ALCOHOL

It has been known for some time that increased alcohol consumption (particularly red wine) is associated with reduced risk for CVD. Alcohol increases HDL-C by: (i) stimulating hepatic Apo A-I secretion and (ii) inhibiting CETP activity. The increase in HDL-C in response to alcohol consumption may in part account for the reduced risk for cardiovascular events among

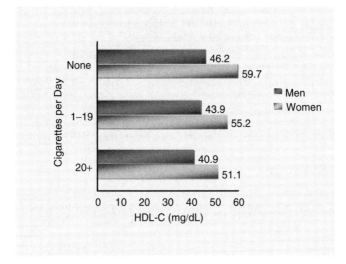

Figure 7.3 Mean serum levels of high-density lipoprotein cholesterol (HDL-C) by cigarette use in the Framingham Offspring Study. Figure kindly provided by Professor Peter W. F. Wilson. Based on Lamon-Fava, S., Wilson, P.W.F. and Schaefer, E.J. (1996) *Arteriosclerosis, Thrombosis, and Vascular Biology*, **16**, 1509–15, [66].

moderate consumers of alcohol. However, alcohol consumption can also increase the serum triglyceride concentration and, in excessive quantities, is associated with increases in various health risks. The relative benefits and risks associated with increased alcohol consumption is an issue that would have to be weighed on a patient by patient basis.

7.7   PHARMACOLOGIC MANAGEMENT OF LOW HDL

The discovery of novel drugs and biomolecules to increase serum levels of HDL-C constitutes a substantial focus in contemporary cardiovascular medicine. The capacity of currently available medications to raise HDL-C is summarized in Table 7.3. The statins, fibrates, and niacin have been shown to favorably impact on cardiovascular morbidity in patients with low HDL-C, though the relative contribution to overall benefit of raising HDL-C has been challenging to elucidate given the fact that all of these medications impact on multiple lipoprotein fractions. A flow chart

Table 7.3 Expected increase in serum high-density cholesterol (HDL-C) in response to various pharmacologic therapies.

Drug	% increase in HDL-C
Statins	3–15
Fibrates	10–15
Niacin	10–30
Thiazolidinediones	5–24
Estrogen	10–25

Taken from National Cholesterol Education Program (2002) Final Report, NIH Publication No. 02-5215, [37].

summarizing possible approaches to the clinical management of low HDL-C is shown in Figure 7.4.

STATINS

The statins or hydroxymethylglutaryl coenzyme A inhibitors impact the metabolism of all hepatically derived lipoproteins, including HDL. The statins impact HDL levels by: (i) stimulating hepatic Apo A-I secretion and (ii) decreasing serum triglycerides, thereby reducing lipolysis and catabolism by HL. The statins increase HDL-C by 3–15%, depending upon their dose and baseline patient characteristics [81, 82]. Patients with hypertriglyceridemia tend to experience larger increases in HDL-C in response to statin therapy than patients with normal levels of triglycerides [83].

Statins should be used as first-line therapy in patients with either isolated low HDL-C or low HDL-C combined with LDL-C that exceeds risk-defined NCEP targets. Statins appear to benefit patients disproportionately with low HDL-C. In one primary prevention study, statin therapy reduced risk for cardiovascular events three-fold more in patients with HDL-C <40 mg dl^{-1} compared with patients whose HDL-C was higher than this threshold [84]. In an angiographic subgroup analysis from the Lipoprotein and Coronary Atherosclerosis Study, patients with HDL-C <35 mg dl^{-1} and treated with fluvastatin experienced significant slowing in the rate of coronary atherosclerosis progression, whereas among patients with HDL ≥35 mg dl^{-1} there was no significant impact on rates of disease progression [85]. In the Heart Protection Study, there was a trend toward increasing benefit with statin therapy as baseline HDL-C decreased [86]. Among elderly patients aged ≥70 years treated with pravastatin, only patients with LDL-C >159 mg dl^{-1} or HDL <43 mg d^{-1} derived significant reductions in cardiovascular events [87].

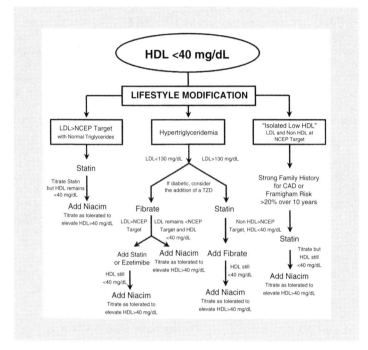

Figure 7.4   Algorithm for treatment of low serum high-density lipoprotein cholesterol (HDL-C). TZD = thiazolidinedione. Reproduced with permission from Toth, P.P. (2004) *Circulation*, **109**, 1809–12, [40] Lippincott Williams & Wilkins.

FIBRATES

Fibrates are synthetic peroxisomal proliferator-activated receptor-α (PPAR-α) agonists that favorably affect both triglyceride and HDL metabolism. Like the statins, fibrates stimulate hepatic Apo A-I expression. Their effect on triglyceride metabolism, however, differs from that of the statins. The fibrates decrease the expression of Apo CIII and increase the expression of Apo CII, which are an inhibitor and activator of lipoprotein lipase, respectively. Consequently, the fibrates increase lipoprotein lipase activity and promote triglyceride and VLDL catabolism. This will result in greater surface coat transfer from large lipoproteins into HDL and reduced catabolism of HDL secondary to decreased enrichment with triglycerides.

In two major trials (Helsinki Heart Study and Bezafibrate Infarction Prevention Study), the fibrates were shown to particularly benefit patients with high triglycerides and low HDL-C [88, 89]. The Veterans Administration High-Density Lipoprotein Intervention Trial (VA-HIT) was the first prospective clinical trial to demonstrate that cardiovascular events could be reduced significantly with a 6% elevation in HDL-C independent of any reduction in serum LDL-C in men with CAD and low baseline HDL-C (mean of 31 mg dl^{-1}) using gemfibrozil [90]. In the Bezafibrate Infarction Prevention trial, patients with CAD were randomized to bezafibrate versus placebo. In this study, coronary mortality decreased by 27% for every 5 mg dl^{-1} rise in HDL-C induced by bezafibrate therapy [91]. Bezafibrate is not yet approved for use in the USA.

When instituting fibrate therapy it is not unusual to observe a rise in serum LDL-C, though this is less frequent with fenofibrate. This occurs secondary to increased conversion of VLDL to LDL in patients with hypertriglyceridemia. The use of gemfibrozil in combination with statins or ezetimibe is not encouraged. Gemfibrozil can block the glucuronidation of the statins, which can lead to increased risk for adverse events such as rhabdomyolysis [92]. Similarly, ezetimibe has some dependence on glucuronidation for elimination. Fenofibrate is a safer alternative to gemfibrozil as it does not adversely impact glucuronidation. It is not yet clear if the addition of a fibrate to a statin further reduces risk for cardiovascular morbidity and mortality. Studies are underway to evaluate this issue more fully in a randomized prospective manner [93]. However, combination therapy can increase the likelihood that a given patient will meet NCEP defined LDL-C and non-HDL-C targets and have significant elevation in HDL-C.

NIACIN

Niacin is a B vitamin and mechanistically is a fascinating drug. Niacin increases HDL-C in a dose-dependent manner according to multiple mechanisms. Niacin decreases holoparticle uptake by hepatocytes by interfering with the activity of the F1 receptor discussed above. Another mechanism was recently elucidated. Niacin binds to another type of receptor in adipose tissue known as *HM74A* [94]. When niacin binds to this receptor, it inhibits the activity of hormone sensitive lipase, an enzyme that hydrolyzes triglycerides to glycerol and free fatty acids. This decreases the amount of free fatty acid entering the portal circulation and liver. This results in lower hepatic VLDL secretion and decreased availability of triglycerides in serum, which will indirectly lead to less catabolism of HDL by HL. At the level of the macrophage, niacin has been shown to increase the expression of ABCA1, which may increase the capacity for Apo A-I and ndHDL lipidation and speciation [95].

In the Coronary Drug Project, niacin was shown to reduce risk for MI and stroke by 27 and 24%, respectively [96]. When used in combination with a statin in patients with CAD, niacin significantly augments risk reduction for cardiovascular events [97] and has been shown to stabilize carotid intima-media thickness measurements [98]. Niacin potentiates the production of prostaglandin D_2, a potent vasodilator that can induce uncomfortable flushing and itching. Taking a 325 mg tablet of aspirin or 600 mg of ibuprofen one hour before taking niacin can reduce the intensity of this flushing secondary to the inhibition of cyclooxygenase. Avoiding spices and alcohol and ingesting niacin with a low fat snack to slow absorption also reduce the risk for flushing. It is recommended that Niaspan (Abbott Pharmaceuticals) be used for the treatment of dyslipidemia. Over the counter preparations of niacin may lack uniform purity and can be associated with significant toxicity.

THIAZOLIDENEDIONES

The thiazolidenediones (TZDs) are PPAR-γ agonists that sensitize peripheral tissue such as skeletal muscle and adipose tissue to insulin. By relieving insulin resistance, the TZDs can induce reductions in serum triglycerides, decrease the conversion of large buoyant LDL to its small dense variant, and increase serum levels of HDL-C. In diabetic patients with dyslipidemia, TZD therapy can significantly augment the effect of lipid-lowering drugs when trying to normalize serum lipoprotein concentrations [99]. The TZDs do not have an indication for use in patients without diabetes.

ESTROGEN

Both endogenous and exogenous estrogens increase HDL-C. The estrogens stimulate hepatic Apo A-I secretion and decrease HL activity [100, 101]. Postmenopausal hormone therapy is not indicated for the treatment of low HDL-C nor to decrease risk for CVD in women. One clinical situation where estrogen may be useful is in a peri- or postmenopausal woman who is symptomatic from estrogen withdrawal. Hormone therapy will likely reduce the intensity of her menopausal symptoms and can also raise her HDL-C if it is low. On the other hand, hormone therapy is also associated with increased serum triglycerides and C-reactive protein levels.

CONTROVERSY

DO WE NEED HDL TREATMENT GOALS?

Given the strong evidence that higher HDL-C and HDL particle number are associated with reduced CHD event risk, the potential usefulness of HDL-related treatment targets is often discussed. In fact, the American Diabetes Association recommends that the HDL-C level should be maintained at a value >40 (men) or >50 (women) mg dl^{-1} for patients with type 2 diabetes [1]. The NCEP ATP III has not recommended a specific HDL-related treatment goal, although they do consider HDL-C a potential target for therapy after treatment goals for LDL-C and non-HDL-C have been achieved. They also advocate the use of non-drug and drug therapies that raise HDL-C levels as part of the management of other lipid and non-lipid risk factors.

There are two main reasons that the NCEP ATP III chose not to establish HDL treatment targets. First, the therapeutic options available to markedly raise HDL-C are limited. With the exception of niacin, which may raise HDL-C by as much as 35%, most lipid altering therapies raise HDL or HDL-C by only 5–15%. Therefore, the available armamentarium for lowering atherogenic lipoproteins is larger and more efficacious than that for raising potentially antiatherogenic lipoproteins.

The second, and more important, reason that the NCEP ATP III elected not to establish HDL-related targets is that the available data have not provided unequivocal support for the efficacy of raising HDL *per se* for lowering event risk. Data from trials in which HDL has been altered with drugs such as statins, fibrates and niacin provides suggestive evidence for a role of HDL elevation in the associated event reduction. However, since these trials altered multiple lipid fractions, and changes in HDL are strongly correlated with changes in other lipoproteins, the independent effect of raising HDL particle number or HDL-C concentration remains uncertain. Furthermore, the metabolism of HDL-C is complex and HDL particle number and/or HDL-C concentration can be modified through a number of mechanisms. At present it is unclear whether all methods whereby the circulating HDL or HDL-C concentration could be raised will be equally effective for lowering CHD event risk.

Two types of HDL-raising drug therapies have proven disappointing with regard to their CHD protective effects. Postmenopausal estrogen therapy raises the HDL-C level by 10–15%, but at least one type of oral estrogen product (conjugated equine estrogens, which were co-administered with medroxyprogesterone acetate for women with intact uteri) has not been found to offer CHD protection in large trials [2–5]. A class of HDL-raising compounds, the cholesteryl ester transfer protein inhibitors, is currently in development and designed to produce large increases in the HDL-C concentration. Unfortunately, the development of the first drug in this class to reach late-stage trials (torcetrapib) was stopped due to worse clinical outcomes among subjects taking the active compound versus placebo [6]. The drug produced impressive alterations in the serum lipid profile (HDL-C increased by 72% and LDL-C declined by 25%), but cardiovascular events and all-cause mortality were higher than in the placebo group, requiring the discontinuation of a large outcomes trial after mean follow-up of 18 months. However, the drug also induced increases in blood pressure and circulating levels of aldosterone, as well as lower serum potassium. It is not clear whether a drug in the same class with similar lipid effects, but lacking the adverse effects on these variables might have the favorable effects on cardiovascular outcomes. Other pharmaceutical companies are proceeding cautiously with the development of other compounds in this class. In addition, other classes of medication primarily intended to alter HDL metabolism are in early stage development.

The authors share the concerns of the NCEP ATP III regarding the usefulness of treatment goals for HDL-C. Therefore, in the absence of additional data showing the efficacy of raising HDL-C for event reduction, we agree that the primary focus should remain on lowering atherogenic lipoproteins, with HDL-C elevation being a secondary objective.

REFERENCES

[1] American Diabetes Association (2008) Position statement: standards of medical care in diabetes – 2008. *Diabetes Care*, **31**, S12–S54.

[2] Manson, J.E., Hsia, J., Johnson, K.C. *et al*. Women's Health Initiative Investigators (2003) Estrogen plus progestin and the risk of coronary heart disease. *The New England Journal of Medicine*, **349**, 523–34.

[3] Hsia, J., Langer, R.D., Manson, J.E. *et al*. Women's Health Initiative Investigators (2006) Conjugated equine estrogens and coronary heart disease: the Women's Health Initiative. *Archives of Internal Medicine*, **166**, 357–65. Erratum in: (2006) *Archives of Internal Medicine*, **10**, 759.

[4] Anderson, G.L., Limacher, M., Assaf, A.R. *et al*. Women's Health Initiative Steering Committee (2004) Effects of conjugated equine estrogen in postmenopausal women with hysterectomy: the Women's Health Initiative randomized controlled trial. *The Journal of the American Medical Association*, **291**, 1701–12.

[5] Hulley, S., Grady, D., Bush, T. *et al*. Heart and Estrogen/Progestin Replacement Study Research Group (1998) Randomized trial of estrogen

plus progestin for secondary prevention of coronary heart disease in post-menopausal women. *The Journal of the American Medical Association*, **280**, 605–13.
[6] Barter, P.J., Caulfield, M., Eriksson, M. *et al*. ILLUMINATE Investigators (2007) Effects of torcetrapib in patients at high risk for coronary events. *The New England Journal of Medicine*, **357**, 2109–22.

REFERENCES

[1] Barr, D.P., Russ, E.M. and Eder, H.A. (1951) Protein-lipid relationships in human plasma. II. In atherosclerosis and related conditions. *The American Journal of Medicine*, **11**, 480–93.

[2] Anderson, G.L., Limacher, M., Assaf, A.R. *et al*. (2004) Effects of conjugated equine estrogen in postmenopausal women with hysterectomy: the Women's Health Initiative randomized controlled trial. *The Journal of the American Medical Association*, **291**, 1701–12.

[3] Weverling-Rijnsburger, A.W., Jonkers, I.J., van Exel, E. *et al*. (2003) High-density vs low-density lipoprotein cholesterol as the risk factor for coronary artery disease and stroke in old age. *Archives of Internal Medicine*, **163**, 1549–54.

[4] Pearson, T.A., Bulkley, B.H., Achuff, S.C. *et al*. (1979) The association of low levels of HDL cholesterol and arteriographically defined coronary artery disease. *American Journal of Epidemiology*, **109**, 285–95.

[5] Shah, P.K. and Amin, J. (1992) Low high-density lipoprotein level is associated with increased restenosis rate after coronary angioplasty. *Circulation*, **85**, 1279–85.

[6] Rizzo, M., Pernice, V., Frasheri, A. and Berneis, K. (2008) Atherogenic lipoprotein phenotype and LDL size and subclasses in patients with peripheral arterial disease. *Atherosclerosis*, **197**, 237–41.

[7] Burke, A.P., Farb, A., Malcom, G.T. *et al*. (1999) Plaque rupture and sudden death related to exertion in men with coronary artery disease. *The Journal of the American Medical Association*, **281**, 921–26.

[8] Castelli, W.P., Garrison, R.J., Wilson, P.W. *et al*. (1986) Incidence of coronary heart disease and lipoprotein cholesterol levels. The Framingham Study. *The Journal of the American Medical Association*, **256**, 2835–38.

[9] Castelli, W.P. (1988) Cholesterol and lipids in the risk of coronary artery disease – the Framingham Heart Study. *The Canadian Journal of Cardiology*, **4** (Suppl A), 5A–10A.

[10] Castelli, W.P., Doyle, J.T., Gordon, T. *et al*. (1977) HDL cholesterol and other lipids in coronary heart disease. The Cooperative Lipoprotein Phenotyping Study. *Circulation*, **55**, 767–72.

[11] Stampfer, M.J., Sacks, F.M., Salvini, S. *et al*. (1991) A prospective study of cholesterol, apolipoproteins, and the risk of myocardial infarction. *The New England Journal of Medicine*, **325**, 373–81.

[12] Miller, N.E., Thelle, D.S., Forde, O.H. and Mjos, O.D. (1977) The Tromso Heart Study: high-density lipoprotein and coronary heart disease: a prospective case-control study. *Lancet*, **1**, 965–68.

[13] Assmann, G., Cullen, P. and Schulte, H. (1998) The Munster Heart Study (PROCAM). Results of follow-up at 8 years. *European Heart Journal*, **19** (Suppl A), A2–A11.

[14] Luc, G., Bard, J.M., Ferrieres, J. *et al*. (2002) Value of HDL cholesterol, apolipoprotein A-I, lipoprotein A-I, and lipoprotein A-I/A-II in prediction of coronary heart disease: the PRIME Study. Prospective Epidemiological Study of Myocardial Infarction. *Arteriosclerosis, Thrombosis, and Vascular Biology*, **22**, 1155–61.

[15] Walldius, G., Jungner, I., Holme, I. *et al*. (2001) High apolipoprotein B, low apolipoprotein A-I, and improvement in the prediction of fatal myocardial infarction (AMORIS Study): a prospective study. *Lancet*, **358**, 2026–33.

[16] Sacco, R.L., Benson, R.T., Kargman, D.E. *et al*. (2001) High-density lipoprotein cholesterol and ischemic stroke in the elderly: the Northern Manhattan Stroke Study. *The Journal of the American Medical Association*, **285**, 2729–35.

[17] Psaty, B.M., Anderson, M., Kronmal, R.A. *et al*. (2004) The association between lipid levels and the risks of incident myocardial infarction, stroke, and total mortality: the Cardiovascular Health Study. *Journal of the American Geriatrics Society*, **52**, 1639–47.

[18] Kitamura, A., Iso, H., Naito, Y. *et al*. (1994) High-density lipoprotein cholesterol and premature coronary heart disease in urban Japanese men. *Circulation*, **89**, 2533–39.

[19] Gordon, D.J., Probstfield, J.L., Garrison, R.J. *et al*. (1989) High-density lipoprotein cholesterol and cardiovascular disease. Four prospective American studies. *Circulation*, **79**, 8–15.

[20] Asztalos, B.F., Cupples, L.A., Demissie, S. *et al*. (2004) High-density lipoprotein subpopulation profile and coronary heart disease prevalence in male participants of the Framingham Offspring Study. *Arteriosclerosis, Thrombosis, and Vascular Biology*, **24**, 2181–87.

[21] Shai, I., Rimm, E.B., Hankinson, S.E. *et al*. (2004) Multivariate assessment of lipid parameters as predictors of coronary heart disease among postmenopausal women: potential implications for clinical guidelines. *Circulation*, **110**, 2824–30.

[22] Wolfram, R.M., Brewer, H.B., Xue, Z. *et al*. (2006) Impact of low high-density lipoproteins on in-hospital events and one-year clinical outcomes in patients with non-ST-elevation myocardial infarction acute coronary syndrome treated with drug-eluting stent implantation. *The American Journal of Cardiology*, **98**, 711–17.

[23] Nicholls, S.J., Tuzcu, E.M., Sipahi, I. *et al*. (2007) Statins, high-density lipoprotein cholesterol, and regression of coronary atherosclerosis. *The Journal of the American Medical Association*, **297**, 499–508.

[24] Ishikawa, K., Tani, S., Watanabe, I. *et al*. (2003) Effect of pravastatin on coronary plaque volume. *The American Journal of Cardiology*, **92**, 975–77.

[25] Expert Panel on Detection, Evaluation and Treatment of High Blood Cholesterol in Adults (2001) Executive summary of the third report of the National Cholesterol Education Program (NCEP) Expert Panel on Detection,

Evaluation, and Treatment of High Blood Cholesterol in Adults (Adult Treatment Panel III). *The Journal of the American Medical Association*, **285**, 2486–97.

[26] Mosca, L., Appel, L.J., Benjamin, E.J. *et al*. (2004) Evidence-based guidelines for cardiovascular disease prevention in women. American Heart Association scientific statement. *Arteriosclerosis, Thrombosis, and Vascular Biology*, **24**, e29–e50.

[27] Ford, E.S., Giles, W.H. and Dietz, W.H. (2002) Prevalence of the metabolic syndrome among US adults: findings from the third National Health and Nutrition Examination Survey. *The Journal of the American Medical Association*, **287**, 356–59.

[28] Sempos, C.T., Cleeman, J.I., Carroll, M.D. *et al*. (1993) Prevalence of high blood cholesterol among US adults. An update based on guidelines from the second report of the National Cholesterol Education Program Adult Treatment Panel. *The Journal of the American Medical Association*, **269**, 3009–14.

[29] Alsheikh-Ali, A.A., Lin, J.L., Abourjaily, P. *et al*. (2007) Prevalence of low high-density lipoprotein cholesterol in patients with documented coronary heart disease or risk equivalent and controlled low-density lipoprotein cholesterol. *The American Journal of Cardiology*, **100**, 1499–501.

[30] Bruckert, E., Baccara-Dinet, M., McCoy, F. and Chapman, J. (2005) High prevalence of low HDL-cholesterol in a pan-European survey of 8545 dyslipidaemic patients. *Current Medical Research and Opinion*, **21**, 1927–34.

[31] Rubins, H.B., Robins, S.J., Collins, D. *et al*. (1995) Distribution of lipids in 8,500 men with coronary artery disease. Department of Veterans Affairs HDL Intervention Trial Study Group. *The American Journal of Cardiology*, **75**, 1196–201.

[32] Schwiesow, S.J., Nappi, J.M. and Ragucci, K.R. (2006) Assessment of compliance with lipid guidelines in an academic medical center. *The Annals of Pharmacotherapy*, **40**, 27–31.

[33] Genest, J. Jr, McNamara, J.R., Ordovas, J.M. *et al*. (1992) Lipoprotein cholesterol, apolipoprotein A-I and B and lipoprotein (a) abnormalities in men with premature coronary artery disease. *Journal of the American College of Cardiology*, **19**, 792–802.

[34] Haffner, S.M. (2004) Dyslipidemia management in adults with diabetes. *Diabetes Care*, **27** (Suppl 1), S68–S71.

[35] Sacks, F.M. (2002) The role of high-density lipoprotein (HDL) cholesterol in the prevention and treatment of coronary heart disease: expert group recommendations. *The American Journal of Cardiology*, **90**, 139–43.

[36] Chapman, M.J., Assmann, G., Fruchart, J.C. *et al*. (2004) Raising high-density lipoprotein cholesterol with reduction of cardiovascular risk: the role of nicotinic acid – position paper developed by the European Consensus Panel on HDL-C. *Current Medical Research and Opinion*, **20**, 1253–68.

[37] National Cholesterol Education Program, National Heart, Lung, and Blood Institute, National Institutes of Health (2002) Third Report of the National Cholesterol Education Program (NCEP) Expert Panel on Detection, Evaluation, and Treatment of High Blood Cholesterol in Adults (Adult Treatment Panel III), Final Report, NIH Publication No. 02-5215.

[38] Toth, P.P. (2001) High-density lipoprotein: epidemiology, metabolism, and antiatherogenic effects. *Disease-a-Month: DM*, **47**, 369–416.

[39] Toth, P.P. (2003) Reverse cholesterol transport: high-density lipoprotein's magnificent mile. *Current Atherosclerosis Reports*, **5**, 386–93.

[40] Toth, P.P. (2004) High-density lipoprotein and cardiovascular risk. *Circulation*, **109**, 1809–12.

[41] Toth, P.P. (2007) Torcetrapib and atherosclerosis: what happened and where do we go from here? *Future Lipidology*, **2**, 277–84.

[42] Brooks-Wilson, A., Marcil, M., Clee, S.M. *et al.* (1999) Mutations in ABC1 in Tangier disease and familial high-density lipoprotein deficiency. *Nature Genetics*, **22**, 336–45.

[43] Vaisman, B.L., Lambert, G., Amar, M. *et al.* (2001) ABCA1 overexpression leads to hyperalphalipoproteinemia and increased biliary cholesterol excretion in transgenic mice. *The Journal of Clinical Investigation*, **108**, 303–9.

[44] Attie, A.D., Kastelein, J.P. and Hayden, M.R. (2001) Pivotal role of ABCA1 in reverse cholesterol transport influencing HDL levels and susceptibility to atherosclerosis. *Journal of Lipid Research*, **42**, 1717–26.

[45] Hovingh, G.K., Brownlie, A., Bisoendial, R.J. *et al.* (2004) A novel apoA-I mutation (L178P) leads to endothelial dysfunction, increased arterial wall thickness, and premature coronary artery disease. *Journal of the American College of Cardiology*, **44**, 1429–35.

[46] Krieger, M. (1999) Charting the fate of the "good cholesterol": identification and characterization of the high-density lipoprotein receptor SR-BI. *Annual Review of Biochemistry*, **68**, 523–58.

[47] Martinez, L.O., Jacquet, S., Esteve, J.P. *et al.* (2003) Ectopic beta-chain of ATP synthase is an apolipoprotein A-I receptor in hepatic HDL endocytosis. *Nature*, **421**, 75–79.

[48] Eriksson, M., Carlson, L.A., Miettinen, T.A. and Angelin, B. (1999) Stimulation of fecal steroid excretion after infusion of recombinant proapolipoprotein A-I. Potential reverse cholesterol transport in humans. *Circulation*, **100**, 594–98.

[49] Naik, S.U., Wang, X., Da Silva, J.S. *et al.* (2006) Pharmacological activation of liver X receptors promotes reverse cholesterol transport in vivo. *Circulation*, **113**, 90–97.

[50] Ramet, M.E., Ramet, M., Lu, Q. *et al.* (2003) High-density lipoprotein increases the abundance of eNOS protein in human vascular endothelial cells by increasing its half-life. *Journal of the American College of Cardiology*, **41**, 2288–97.

[51] Levkau, B., Hermann, S., Theilmeier, G. *et al.* (2004) High-density lipoprotein stimulates myocardial perfusion in vivo. *Circulation*, **110**, 3355–59.

[52] Xia, P., Vadas, M.A., Rye, K.A. *et al.* (1999) High-density lipoproteins (HDL) interrupt the sphingosine kinase signaling pathway. A possible mechanism for protection against atherosclerosis by HDL. *The Journal of Biological Chemistry*, **274**, 33143–47.

[53] Kimura, T., Sato, K., Malchinkhuu, E. *et al.* (2003) High-density lipoprotein stimulates endothelial cell migration and survival through sphingosine 1-phosphate and its receptors. *Arteriosclerosis, Thrombosis, and Vascular Biology*, **23**, 1283–88.

[54] Aviram, M., Hardak, E., Vaya, J. *et al.* (2000) Human serum paraoxonases (PON1) Q and R selectively decrease lipid peroxides in human coronary and carotid atherosclerotic lesions: PON1 esterase and peroxidase-like activities. *Circulation*, **101**, 2510–17.

[55] Stremler, K.E., Stafforini, D.M., Prescott, S.M. and McIntyre, T.M. (1991) Human plasma platelet-activating factor acetylhydrolase. Oxidatively fragmented phospholipids as substrates. *The Journal of Biological Chemistry*, **266**, 11095–103.

[56] Vinals, M., Martinez-Gonzalez, J. and Badimon, L. (1999) Regulatory effects of HDL on smooth muscle cell prostacyclin release. *Arteriosclerosis, Thrombosis, and Vascular Biology*, **19**, 2405–11.

[57] Nofer, J.R., Walter, M., Kehrel, B. *et al.* (1998) HDL3-mediated inhibition of thrombin-induced platelet aggregation and fibrinogen binding occurs via decreased production of phosphoinositide-derived second messengers 1,2-diacylglycerol and inositol 1,4,5-tris-phosphate. *Arteriosclerosis, Thrombosis, and Vascular Biology*, **18**, 861–69.

[58] Griffin, J.H., Kojima, K., Banka, C.L. *et al.* (1999) High-density lipoprotein enhancement of anticoagulant activities of plasma protein S and activated protein C. *The Journal of Clinical Investigation*, **103**, 219–27.

[59] Beitz, J. and Mest, H.J. (1986) Thromboxane A2 (TXA2) formation by washed human platelets under the influence of low and high-density lipoproteins from healthy donors. *Prostaglandins, Leukotrienes, and Medicine*, **23**, 303–9.

[60] Miyazaki, A., Sakuma, S., Morikawa, W. *et al.* (1995) Intravenous injection of rabbit apolipoprotein A-I inhibits the progression of atherosclerosis in cholesterol-fed rabbits. *Arteriosclerosis, Thrombosis, and Vascular Biology*, **15**, 1882–88.

[61] Tangirala, R.K., Tsukamoto, K., Chun, S.H. *et al.* (1999) Regression of atherosclerosis induced by liver-directed gene transfer of apolipoprotein A-I in mice. *Circulation*, **100**, 1816–22.

[62] Badimon, J.J., Badimon, L. and Fuster, V. (1990) Regression of atherosclerotic lesions by high-density lipoprotein plasma fraction in the cholesterol-fed rabbit. *The Journal of Clinical Investigation*, **85**, 1234–41.

[63] Tardif, J.C., Gregoire, J., L'Allier, P.L. *et al.* (2007) Effects of reconstituted high-density lipoprotein infusions on coronary atherosclerosis: a randomized controlled trial. *The Journal of the American Medical Association*, **297**, 1675–82.

[64] Badellino, K.O. and Rader, D.J. (2004) The role of endothelial lipase in high-density lipoprotein metabolism. *Current Opinion in Cardiology*, **19**, 392–95.

[65] Duong, M., Psaltis, M., Rader, D.J. *et al.* (2003) Evidence that hepatic lipase and endothelial lipase have different substrate specificities for high-density lipoprotein phospholipids. *Biochemistry*, **42**, 13778–85.

[66] Lamon-Fava, S., Wilson, P.W.F. and Schaefer, E.J. (1996) Impact of body mass index on coronary heart disease risk factors in men and women. The Framingham Offspring Study. *Arteriosclerosis, Thrombosis, and Vascular Biology*, **16**, 1509–15.

[67] Dattilo, A.M. and Kris-Etherton, P.M. (1992) Effects of weight reduction on blood lipids and lipoproteins: a meta-analysis. *The American Journal of Clinical Nutrition*, **56**, 320–28.

[68] Berglund, L., Oliver, E.H., Fontanez, N. *et al.* (1999) HDL-subpopulation patterns in response to reductions in dietary total and saturated fat intakes in healthy subjects. *The American Journal of Clinical Nutrition*, **70**, 992–1000.

[69] Appel, L.J., Sacks, F.M., Carey, V.J. *et al.* (2005) Effects of protein, monounsaturated fat, and carbohydrate intake on blood pressure and serum lipids: results of the OmniHeart randomized trial. *The Journal of the American Medical Association*, **294**, 2455–64.

[70] Dansinger, M.L., Gleason, J.A., Griffith, J.L. *et al.* (2005) Comparison of the Atkins, Ornish, Weight Watchers, and Zone diets for weight loss and heart disease risk reduction: a randomized trial. *The Journal of the American Medical Association*, **293**, 43–53.

[71] Matthan, N.R., Welty, F.K., Barrett, P.H. *et al.* (2004) Dietary hydrogenated fat increases high-density lipoprotein apoA-I catabolism and decreases low-density lipoprotein apoB-100 catabolism in hypercholesterolemic women. *Arteriosclerosis, Thrombosis, and Vascular Biology*, **24**, 1092–97.

[72] Esposito, K., Marfella, R., Ciotola, M. *et al.* (2004) Effect of a mediterranean-style diet on endothelial dysfunction and markers of vascular inflammation in the metabolic syndrome: a randomized trial. *The Journal of the American Medical Association*, **292**, 1440–46.

[73] Kokkinos, P.F. and Fernhall, B. (1999) Physical activity and high-density lipoprotein cholesterol levels: what is the relationship? *Sports Medicine*, **28**, 307–14.

[74] Kokkinos, P.F., Holland, J.C., Narayan, P. *et al.* (1995) Miles run per week and high-density lipoprotein cholesterol levels in healthy, middle-aged men. A dose-response relationship. *Archives of Internal Medicine*, **155**, 415–20.

[75] Welty, F.K., Stuart, E., O'Meara, M. and Huddleston, J. (2002) Effect of addition of exercise to therapeutic lifestyle changes diet in enabling women and men with coronary heart disease to reach Adult Treatment Panel III low-density lipoprotein cholesterol goal without lowering high-density lipoprotein cholesterol. *The American Journal of Cardiology*, **89**, 1201–4.

[76] Couillard, C., Despres, J.P., Lamarche, B. *et al.* (2001) Effects of endurance exercise training on plasma HDL cholesterol levels depend on levels of triglycerides: evidence from men of the Health, Risk Factors, Exercise Training and Genetics (HERITAGE) Family Study. *Arteriosclerosis, Thrombosis, and Vascular Biology*, **21**, 1226–32.

[77] Garrison, R.J., Kannel, W.B., Feinleib, M. *et al.* (1978) Cigarette smoking and HDL cholesterol: the Framingham Offspring Study. *Atherosclerosis*, **30**, 17–25.

[78] Cullen, P., Schulte, H. and Assmann, G. (1998) Smoking, lipoproteins and coronary heart disease risk. Data from the Munster Heart Study (PROCAM). *European Heart Journal*, **19**, 1632–41.

[79] Imamura, H., Teshima, K., Miyamoto, N. and Shirota, T. (2002) Cigarette smoking, high-density lipoprotein cholesterol subfractions, and lecithin: cholesterol acyltransferase in young women. *Metabolism: Clinical and Experimental*, **51**, 1313–16.

[80] Moffatt, R.J. (1990) Normalization of high-density lipoprotein cholesterol following cessation from cigarette smoking. *Advances in Experimental Medicine and Biology*, **273**, 267–72.

152HDL CHOLESTEROL

[81] Jones, P.H., Davidson, M.H., Stein, E.A. *et al.* (2003) Comparison of the efficacy and safety of rosuvastatin versus atorvastatin, simvastatin, and pravastatin across doses (STELLAR* Trial). *The American Journal of Cardiology*, **92**, 152–60.

[82] Nissen, S.E., Nicholls, S.J., Sipahi, I. *et al.* (2006) Effect of very high-intensity statin therapy on regression of coronary atherosclerosis: the ASTEROID trial. *The Journal of the American Medical Association*, **295**, 1556–65.

[83] Crouse, J.R. III, Frohlich, J., Ose, L. *et al.* (1999) Effects of high doses of simvastatin and atorvastatin on high-density lipoprotein cholesterol and apolipoprotein A-I. *The American Journal of Cardiology*, **83**, 1476–77, A1477.

[84] Downs, J.R., Clearfield, M., Weis, S. *et al.* (1998) Primary prevention of acute coronary events with lovastatin in men and women with average cholesterol levels: results of AFCAPS/TexCAPS. Air Force/Texas Coronary Atherosclerosis Prevention Study. *The Journal of the American Medical Association*, **279**, 1615–22.

[85] Ballantyne, C.M., Herd, J.A., Ferlic, L.L. *et al.* (1999) Influence of low HDL on progression of coronary artery disease and response to fluvastatin therapy. *Circulation*, **99**, 736–43.

[86] Heart Protection Study Collaborative Group (2002) MRC/BHF Heart Protection Study of cholesterol lowering with simvastatin in 20,536 high-risk individuals: a randomised placebo-controlled trial. *Lancet*, **360**, 7–22.

[87] Shepherd, J., Blauw, G.J., Murphy, M.B. *et al.* (2002) Pravastatin in elderly individuals at risk of vascular disease (PROSPER): a randomised controlled trial. *Lancet*, **360**, 1623–30.

[88] Manninen, V., Elo, M.O., Frick, M.H. *et al.* (1988) Lipid alterations and decline in the incidence of coronary heart disease in the Helsinki Heart Study. *The Journal of the American Medical Association*, **260**, 641–51.

[89] BIP Study Group (2000) Secondary prevention by raising HDL cholesterol and reducing triglycerides in patients with coronary artery disease: the Bezafibrate Infarction Prevention (BIP) Study. *Circulation*, **102**, 21–27.

[90] Robins, S.J., Collins, D., Wittes, J.T. *et al.* (2001) Relation of gemfibrozil treatment and lipid levels with major coronary events: VA-HIT: a randomized controlled trial. *The Journal of the American Medical Association*, **285**, 1585–91.

[91] Goldenberg, I., Goldbourt, U., Boyko, V. *et al.* (2006) Relation between on-treatment increments in serum high-density lipoprotein cholesterol levels and cardiac mortality in patients with coronary heart disease (from the Bezafibrate Infarction Prevention trial). *The American Journal of Cardiology*, **97**, 466–71.

[92] Prueksaritanont, T., Zhao, J.J., Ma, B. *et al.* (2002) Mechanistic studies on metabolic interactions between gemfibrozil and statins. *The Journal of Pharmacology and Experimental Therapeutics*, **301**, 1042–51.

[93] Zambon, A. and Cusi, K. (2007) The role of fenofibrate in clinical practice. *Diabetes and Vascular Disease Research*, **4** (Suppl 3), S15–S20.

[94] Tunaru, S., Kero, J., Schaub, A. *et al.* (2003) PUMA-G and HM74 are receptors for nicotinic acid and mediate its anti-lipolytic effect. *Nature Medicine*, **9**, 352–55.

[95] Rubic, T., Trottmann, M. and Lorenz, R.L. (2004) Stimulation of CD36 and the key effector of reverse cholesterol transport ATP-binding cassette A1 in monocytoid cells by niacin. *Biochemical Pharmacology*, **67**, 411–19.

[96] The Coronary Drug Project Research Group (1975) Clofibrate and niacin in coronary heart disease. *The Journal of the American Medical Association*, **231**, 360–81.

[97] Brown, B.G., Zhao, X.Q., Chait, A. *et al.* (2001) Simvastatin and niacin, antioxidant vitamins, or the combination for the prevention of coronary disease. *The New England Journal of Medicine*, **345**, 1583–92.

[98] Taylor, A.J., Sullenberger, L.E., Lee, H.J. *et al.* (2004) Arterial biology for the investigation of the treatment effects of reducing cholesterol (ARBITER) 2: a double-blind, placebo-controlled study of extended-release niacin on atherosclerosis progression in secondary prevention patients treated with statins. *Circulation*, **110**, 3512–17.

[99] Goldberg, R.B., Kendall, D.M., Deeg, M.A. *et al.* (2005) A comparison of lipid and glycemic effects of pioglitazone and rosiglitazone in patients with type 2 diabetes and dyslipidemia. *Diabetes Care*, **28**, 1547–54.

[100] Tikkanen, M.J., Nikkila, E.A., Kuusi, T. and Sipinen, S.U. (1982) High-density lipoprotein-2 and hepatic lipase: reciprocal changes produced by estrogen and norgestrel. *The Journal of Clinical Endocrinology and Metabolism*, **54**, 1113–17.

[101] Jin, F.Y., Kamanna, V.S. and Kashyap, M.L. (1998) Estradiol stimulates apolipoprotein A-I- but not A-II-containing particle synthesis and secretion by stimulating mRNA transcription rate in Hep G2 cells. *Arteriosclerosis, Thrombosis, and Vascular Biology*, **18**, 999–1006.

8 Lipid Management in Population Subsets: Women, the Elderly, Ethnic Minorities, Children, and Adolescents

Key Points

- *Many major coronary heart disease (CHD) risk factors and treatment goals are the same across the population subsets of race, gender, ethnicity, and age, although population surveys show that diagnosis and successful treatment of lipid abnormalities vary substantially across these same subsets.*

- *More US women die of cardiovascular-related deaths than men each year and, fortunately, women have been better represented in recent years in primary and secondary prevention studies of lipid interventions.*

- *Results of the Heart Protection Study (HPS) demonstrated that the relative risk reduction associated with simvastatin therapy was similar in men and women, but the National Cholesterol Education Program Evaluation Program Using Novel E-technology (NEPTUNE) II survey showed that although both sexes had similar frequencies of lipid treatment goal achievement in the low and moderate risk categories, fewer women achieved the goal in the high-risk (CHD and risk equivalents) category.*

- *The National Cholesterol Education Program Adult Treatment Panel (NCEP ATP) III report states that low-density lipoprotein cholesterol (LDL-C) lowering in elderly subjects (≥ 65 years for men and ≥ 75 years for women) should not be denied and lifestyle interventions for lipid management, including a diet low in saturated fats, trans fats,* *and cholesterol, and the increased ingestion of viscous fibers and plant sterol/stanol products, should be encouraged.*

- *Minority populations display high prevalence values for several major risk factors, which, in turn, results in higher rates of cardiovascular events.*

- *A number of surveys show that the major ethnic and racial minority groups in the USA are less likely to receive preventive care and therefore less likely to achieve treatment goals.*

- *Identification and treatment of childhood and adolescent dyslipidemia, especially for high-risk individuals (defined by the NCEP ATP III as family history of a myocardial infarction or sudden death in a first-degree male relative <55 years of age or a first-degree female relative <65 years of age), is an important preventive strategy because atherosclerosis is a lifelong, progressive disease with its origins in preadulthood.*

The NCEP ATP III treatment goals do not differentiate between subgroups within the adult population. Furthermore, major CHD risk factors are largely the same, regardless of gender or ethnicity, although some notable differences exist in the prevalence of specific risk factors among subsets in the population. In addition, population surveys show that diagnosis and successful treatment of lipid abnormalities vary substantially across population subsets. The focus of this chapter will be on special considerations and challenges in the diagnosis and management of dyslipidemias in selected population subsets, including women, the elderly, ethnic minority groups, children, and adolescents.

8.1   WOMEN

CARDIOVASCULAR DISEASE RISK IN WOMEN

Cardiovascular diseases, particularly CHD and stroke, are the leading causes of death among women in the USA. More women than men die in the USA of cardiovascular disease each year and cardiovascular diseases account for more deaths than the next seven causes combined [1]. Surveys have consistently shown that women tend to feel more at risk of death from cancer, particularly breast cancer, than cardiovascular disease, despite the fact that the number of deaths from cardiovascular disease in women each year is more than 10 times that of breast cancer and nearly twice that of all cancers combined [1, 2]. Average lifetime risk for symptomatic cardiovascular disease is roughly 50% for 40-year-old US women [1].

8.2 LIPIDS IN WOMEN

The main difference in the lipid profile between men and women is that the average high-density lipoprotein cholesterol (HDL-C) concentration is ~10 mg dl^{-1} higher in women after puberty. This difference appears to be primarily due to the effects of testosterone to depress the HDL-C concentration in males rather than the effects of endogenous estrogen in females, as is commonly believed [3, 4]. The LDL-C concentration tends to be slightly lower in women than men during the young adult years, but increases in middle age. The increase in LDL-C is larger in women between the ages of 40 and 60 than in men [5]. This is at least partially accounted for by a rise in LDL-C associated with menopause in women [6].

The relationship between LDL-C and relative risk for CHD is similar in men and women. However, disturbances in the levels of triglyceride-rich lipoproteins and HDL-C appear to be more strongly associated with increased risk in women than men. For example, each 1 mg dl^{-1} increment in HDL-C is associated with a 3% reduction in cardiovascular event risk in women, but only a 2% reduction in men. Moreover, diabetes mellitus, which is characterized by disturbances in triglyceride-rich lipoprotein and HDL-C concentrations, accounts for a three- to sevenfold increase in CHD risk in women, compared with a two- to threefold increase in men.

8.3 TREATMENT OF DYSLIPIDEMIA IN WOMEN

Women were underrepresented in early trials of lipid-altering therapies. However, in recent years, substantial numbers of women have been included in both primary and secondary prevention studies of lipid interventions (primarily statin trials). For example, the HPS enrolled 20 536 subjects in the United Kingdom [7]. Women were 25% of the sample. HPS subjects were a combination of those with preexisting atherosclerotic disease (CHD and peripheral arterial disease), individuals with diabetes, and those multiple risk factors that put them at high risk for a cardiovascular event. Figure 8.1 shows results from the HPS by age and sex. The relative risk reduction associated with simvastatin therapy was similar in men and women, as well as for younger and older subjects. These results are representative of those reported for several other large outcome trials and illustrate the efficacy of therapies to lower atherogenic lipoproteins across all major population subgroups.

In the NEPTUNE II survey, women and men had similar frequencies of lipid treatment goal achievement in the low and moderate risk categories, but were significantly less likely to have achieved goal in the high-risk (CHD and risk equivalents) subgroup (Figure 8.2). This suggests that high-risk women may receive less aggressive treatment for dyslipidemia, a practice not supported by the available evidence. Thus, extra vigilance is warranted

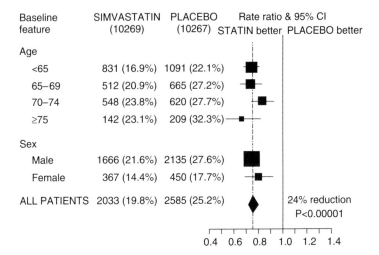

Figure 8.1 Major vascular events in the simvastatin and placebo groups of the Heart Protection Study according to baseline age and sex categories. Reproduced from Collins *et al.* (2002) *Lancet*, **360**, 7–22, [7] with permission from Elsevier.

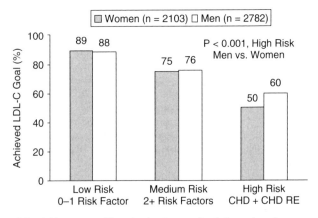

Figure 8.2 Achievement of low-density lipoprotein cholesterol goals among men and women in the National Cholesterol Education Program Evaluation Program Using Novel E-technology (NEPTUNE) II Survey. From Davidson *et al.* (2005) *The American Journal of Cardiology*, **96**, 556–63, [9] with permission of Elsevier.

in clinical practice to identify women at high and very high CHD risk to insure that they are receiving treatment consistent with current guidelines. Additional information regarding prevention of cardiovascular disease in women may be found in the American Heart Association's *Evidence-Based Guidelines for Cardiovascular Disease Prevention in Women: 2007 Update* [8].

8.4 SEX HORMONE THERAPY, LIPIDS, AND CARDIOVASCULAR RISK IN MENOPAUSAL WOMEN

Observational studies over several decades had suggested a beneficial role for estrogen and estrogen/progestin therapy on cardiovascular event risk in women after menopause. Unfortunately, results from three large, randomized, placebo-controlled trials did not support the protective effect suggested by population data [10–12]. For this reason, despite the effects of oral estrogen therapy to reduce LDL-C and raise HDL-C, the National Cholesterol Education Program (NCEP) and the American Heart Association guidelines do not recommend the use of hormone therapy for prevention of cardiovascular disease in women.

8.5 THE ELDERLY

The NCEP ATP III defines elderly as age ≥ 65 years for men and ≥ 75 years for women. The fraction of the US population defined as elderly is increasing rapidly, in part due to advances in medical care that are allowing people to live longer. It is anticipated that the number of people in the USA who are 65 years of age or older will double during the first 30 years of the twenty-first century, increasing from 35 million to over 70 million [13].

While atherosclerosis is a disease that begins in childhood, its consequences (clinical events) are most often experienced in the late-middle age and elderly years. Age is the most powerful risk factor in the Framingham risk equation. However, other major CHD risk factors continue to predict events into the 80s. The relative risk associated with CHD risk factors may diminish somewhat with advanced age, but this is offset by higher absolute risk. Results from large trials show that benefits of reducing LDL-C are evident in the elderly. The relative benefit is similar to, or slightly less than that in middle-aged subjects (for example, see Figure 8.1), but the absolute benefit is greater because of the higher risk for a cardiovascular event in the older patient. Therefore, the NCEP ATP III report states that the benefits of LDL-C lowering should not be denied to elderly subjects strictly on the basis of age [14].

8.6   SPECIAL CONSIDERATIONS FOR LIPID MANAGEMENT IN THE ELDERLY

Elderly patients are often taking multiple medications and pharmacotherapy must be applied with caution to avoid drug interactions that may lead to adverse side effects. Drug clearance may be slower in elderly patients due to reduced renal and hepatic functions, thus increasing susceptibility to side effects of lipid-altering medications. Hypothyroidism is common among the elderly and may be an overlooked factor contributing to hypercholesterolemia. Thyroid hormone replacement will generally improve total cholesterol, LDL-C and triglyceride levels.

Lifestyle interventions for lipid management, including a diet low in saturated fats, *trans* fats and cholesterol, use of viscous fibers and plant sterol/stanol products, and regular physical activity are helpful and effective, but underutilized in the elderly. In particular, physical activity is important for maintaining function and preventing frailty, as well as for its favorable impact on cardiovascular risk factors and event rates.

8.7   ETHNIC MINORITIES

RACIAL/ETHNIC DISPARITIES IN QUANTITY AND QUALITY OF HEALTH CARE

Racial and ethnic disparities in cardiovascular disease event rates and outcomes have been well documented. Minority populations, particularly African Americans, Hispanic/Latino Americans, and Native Americans display high levels of several major CHD risk factors, which appear to account for their increased cardiovascular event rates. For example, in the Atherosclerosis Risk in Communities Study, 80% of African Americans had at least one elevated risk factor, compared with 60% of Whites. After adjustment for risk factor differences and education level, the disparity between the two groups in cardiovascular event rates disappeared [15]. Given the evidence supporting the efficacy of interventions for risk factor modification, particularly treatment of dyslipidemia and hypertension, as well as smoking cessation, it appears likely that intensified efforts to diagnose and treat CHD risk factors could have a major impact on reducing excess cardiovascular morbidity and mortality in these subsets of the population.

A number of surveys have shown that minorities are less likely to receive preventive care, and are less likely to have achieved treatment goals when undergoing risk factor management [9, 16, 17]. Lack of health insurance represents a significant barrier to delivery of preventive healthcare services. Table 8.1 shows the major ethnic groups as percentages of the

Table 8.1 Racial/ethnic breakdown of the US population and uninsured population.

RaceeEthnicity	US population (%)	Uninsured population (%)
Non-Hispanic (Latino) White	69.1	50.2
Latino	12.5	25.8
African American	12.3	17.1
Asian or Pacific Islander	3.3	5.2
American Indian or Alaska Native	0.9	1.8

Adapted from The American College of Physicians Position Statement on Racial and Ethnic Disparities in Healthcare. (2004) *Annals of Internal Medicine*, **141**, 226–32, [16].

US population, as well as the uninsured population. Racial/ethnic minority groups are overrepresented among the uninsured.

Access to health care services does not appear to be the only factor influencing treatment success. In the NEPTUNE II survey, ethnic minorities undergoing lipid management were less likely to have achieved their LDL-C treatment goals than non-Hispanic White subjects (see Figure 8.3) [9, 17]. The relationship of African American versus non-Hispanic White ethnicity on goal achievement remained highly significant after statistical

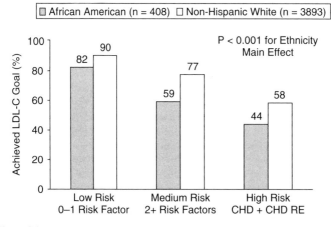

Figure 8.3 Achievement of low-density lipoprotein cholesterol goals among non-Hispanic white and African American subjects in the National Cholesterol Education Program Evaluation Program Using Novel E-technology (NEPTUNE) II Survey. From Clark *et al.* (2006) *Journal of General Internal Medicine*, **21**, 320–26, [17] with permission from Blackwell Publishing.

adjustment for various predictors, including type of treatment prescribed and physician specialty [17]. This suggests that compliance with recommended treatment plans may have been lower, which is in agreement with results from other lines of evidence. The degree to which this might be attributable to differences in income, education level, cultural factors or other causes is not fully understood and deserving of additional research effort. Regardless, physicians should recognize that suboptimal risk factor control is common among ethnic minorities and that this contributes to their higher rates of cardiovascular morbidity and mortality.

8.8   RISK FACTOR INCIDENCE AND PREVALENCE IN ETHNIC MINORITY GROUPS

Several differences in risk factor incidence and prevalence are evident across ethnic groups. Hypertension is more common and has a younger age at onset among African Americans. However, African Americans also have higher average levels of HDL-C and lower triglycerides [1]. Obesity and diabetes are more common among all major ethnic minority groups in the USA than among non-Hispanic Whites [1]. Some Native American groups have exceptionally high prevalences of current smoking [1]. Americans of Asian Indian ethnicity are more likely to have an abdominal visceral pattern of body fat distribution, which may lead to the development of the metabolic syndrome and diabetes at lower body mass index levels than in other ethnic groups [18].

8.9   CHILDREN AND ADOLESCENTS

CHILDHOOD ROOTS OF ATHEROSCLEROSIS

Autopsy studies of young men killed in the Korean and Vietnam wars provided evidence that atherosclerotic disease was present in early adulthood [19, 20]. Subsequent studies of younger boys and girls who died from accidents unrelated to cardiovascular disease confirmed the presence of fatty streaks and atherosclerotic lesions (sometimes advanced lesions) in children and adolescents [21]. Data from the Pathobiological Determinants of Atherosclerosis in Youth and Bogalusa Heart Studies showed that the extent of coronary atherosclerosis in children and adolescents correlated with age, as well as the premortem presence and severity of traditional CHD risk factors, including blood lipids (LDL-C, HDL-C, triglycerides), blood pressure, and body mass index [22]. These data provide evidence that atherosclerosis begins in childhood and is related to the same risk factors that have been identified in adults.

NCEP AND AMERICAN HEART ASSOCIATION RECOMMENDATIONS FOR CHOLESTEROL SCREENING AND MANAGEMENT IN CHILDREN AND ADOLESCENTS

Only one report has been issued by the NCEP regarding cholesterol screening and management in children and adolescents [23]. Additional guidance was issued by the American Heart Association in 2007 [24].

Given evidence supporting the association of dyslipidemia with childhood atherosclerosis, as well as evidence showing that cholesterol levels tend to track from childhood into adulthood (children with high relative cholesterol levels tend to become adults with high relative cholesterol levels), identification and treatment of dyslipidemia in high-risk children and adolescents is an important preventive strategy. The NCEP panel has recommended a targeted approach to screening for lipid abnormalities in children and adolescents. They advise measurement of a lipid profile in cases where a family history exists of either premature cardiovascular disease or elevated blood cholesterol. As discussed in Chapter 3, the NCEP ATP III has defined family history of premature CHD as a myocardial infarction or sudden death in a first-degree male relative <55 years of age or a first-degree female relative <65 years of age. (Note: the authors of this text recommend extending the definition to include other forms of clinically evident atherosclerosis.) Studies evaluating family history of elevated cholesterol or of cardiovascular disease suggest that this would result in the screening of approximately 40% of children and adolescents [25].

Acceptable levels of total and LDL-C are considered to be below the 75th percentile. Levels in the 75th–95th percentiles are considered borderline and those greater than the 95th percentile are considered elevated (Table 8.2). The primary treatment goal is to maintain a LDL-C level less than the 75th percentile, that is, <110 mg dl^{-1}.

Table 8.2 Classifications of total and low-density lipoprotein cholesterol (LDL-C) levels in children and adolescents.

Category	Percentile	Total cholesterol (mg dl^{-1})	LDL-C (mg dl^{-1})
Acceptable	<75th	<170	<110
Borderline	75th–94th	170–199	110–129
Elevated	>95th	≥200	≥130

Adapted from National Cholesterol Education Program Expert Panel on Blood Cholesterol Levels in Children and Adolescents. National Cholesterol Education Program (NCEP): Highlights of the report of the expert panel on blood cholesterol levels in children and adolescents. (1992) *Pediatrics*, **89**, 495–501, [23].

Table 8.3 Recommended values for pharmacologic treatment of children and adolescents ages 10 years and older.

Patient characteristics	Recommended cutpoints
No other major cardiovascular risk factors	LDL-C persistently >190 mg dl^{-1} despite therapeutic lifestyle changes
Other risk factors present including obesity, hypertension, diabetes, smoking, positive family history of premature cardiovascular disease	LDL-C persistently >160 mg dl^{-1} despite therapeutic lifestyle changes

Adapted from National Cholesterol Education Program Expert Panel on Blood Cholesterol Levels in Children and Adolescents. National Cholesterol Education Program (NCEP): Highlights of the report of the Expert Panel on blood cholesterol levels in children and adolescents. (1992) *Pediatrics*, **89**, 495–501, [23].

For children with elevated total and/or LDL-C levels, the general approach to management parallels that for adults: (i) therapeutic lifestyle changes, (ii) use of dietary adjuncts (foods containing sterols/stanols and viscous fibers), and (iii) drug therapy for selected high-risk individuals. Therapeutic lifestyle changes include consumption of a diet low in saturated fat, *trans* fat, and cholesterol for children over two years of age, weight management if overweight or obese, and regular physical activity. Pharmacologic therapy is recommended for selected children and adolescents ages 10 years and above, as outlined in Table 8.3, if a three- to six-month trial of nonpharmacological therapies does not adequately control the LDL-C concentration. The interested reader is referred to the recent American Heart Association Scientific Statement *Drug Therapy of High-risk Lipid Abnormalities in Children and Adolescents* for more information regarding use of drug treatments in patients less than 20 years of age [24].

REFERENCES

[1] American Heart Association (2007) *Heart Disease and Stroke Statistics – 2007 Update*, American Heart Association, Dallas.

[2] Kushi, L.H., Byers, T., Doyle, C. *et al.* The American Cancer Society 2006 Nutrition and Physical Activity Guidelines Advisory Committee (2006) American cancer society guidelines on nutrition and physical activity for cancer prevention: reducing the risk of cancer with healthy food choices and physical activity. *CA: A Cancer Journal for Clinicians*, **56**, 254–81.

[3] Kirkland, R.T., Keenan, B.S., Probstfield, J.L. *et al.* (1987) Decrease in plasma high-density lipoprotein cholesterol levels at puberty in boys with delayed adolescence. *The Journal of the American Medical Association*, **257**, 502–7.

[4] Laskarzewski, P.M., Morrison, J.A., Gutai, J. *et al.* (1983) Longitudinal relationships among endogenous testosterone, estradiol, and Quetelet index with high

REFERENCES

and low density lipoprotein cholesterols in adolescent boys. *Pedia*
17, 689–98.

[5] Carroll, M.D., Lacher, D.A., Sorlie, P.D. *et al.* (2005) Trends in serum lipids and lipoproteins of adults, 1960-2002. *The Journal of the American Medical Association*, **294**, 1773–81.

[6] Meagher, E.A. (2007) Cardiovascular disease in women: the management of dyslipidemia, in *Therapeutic Lipidology*, (eds M.H. Davidson, P.P. Toth and K.C. Maki), Humana Press, Totowa.

[7] Collins, R., Armitage, J., Parish, S. *et al.* (2002) Heart Protection Study Collaborative Group. MRC/BHF Heart Protection Study of cholesterol lowering with simvastatin in 20,536 high risk individuals: a randomised placebo-controlled trial. *Lancet*, **360**, 7–22.

[8] Mosca, L., Banka, C.L., Benjamin, E.J. *et al.* The Expert Panel/Writing Group (2007) Evidence-based guidelines for cardiovascular disease prevention in women: 2007 update. *Circulation*, **115**, 1481–501.

[9] Davidson, M.H., Maki, K.C., Pearson, T.A. *et al.* (2005) Results of the National Cholesterol Education Program (NCEP) Evaluation ProjecT Utilizing Novel E-Technology (NEPTUNE) II survey and implications for treatment under the recent NCEP Writing Group recommendations. *The American Journal of Cardiology*, **96**, 556–63.

[10] Anderson, G.L., Limacher, M., Assaf, A.R. *et al.* (2004) Effects of conjugated equine estrogen in postmenopausal women with hysterectomy: the Women's Health initiative randomized controlled trial. *The Journal of the American Medical Association*, **291**, 1701–12.

[11] Manson, J.E., Hsia, J., Johnson, K.C. *et al.* (2003) Estrogen plus progestin and the risk of coronary heart disease. *The New England Journal of Medicine*, **349**, 523–34.

[12] Writing Group for the Women's Health Initiative Investigators (2002) Risks and benefits of estrogen plus progestin in healthy postmenopausal women: principal results from the Women's Health Initiative randomized controlled trial. *The Journal of the American Medical Association*, **288**, 321–33.

[13] Administration on Aging. U.S. Department of Health and Human Services (2007) (n.d.). A Profile of Older Americans: 2001, http://www.aoa.gov/aoa/stats/profile/2001/2001profile.pdf (accessed on 15 May).

[14] National Cholesterol Education Program. National Heart, Lung, and Blood Institute. National Institutes of Health (2002) *Third Report of the National Cholesterol Education Program (NCEP) Expert Panel on Detection, Evaluation, and Treatment of High Blood Cholesterol in Adults (Adult Treatment Panel III)*, Final Report. NIH Publication No. 02-5215.

[15] Hozawa, A., Folsom, A.R., Sharrett, A.R. and Chambless, L.E. (2007) Absolute and attributable risks of cardiovascular disease incidence in relation to optimal and borderline risk factors: comparison of African American with white subjects – Atherosclerosis Risk in Communities Study. *Archives of Internal Medicine*, **167**, 573–79.

[16] American College of Physicians (2004) Racial and ethnic disparities in health care: a position paper of the American College of Physicians. *Annals of Internal Medicine*, **141**, 226–32.

[17] Clark, L.T., Maki, K.C., Galant, R. *et al.* (2006) Ethnic differences in achievement of cholesterol treatment goals. Results from the National Cholesterol Education Program Evaluation Project Utilizing Novel E-Technology II. *Journal of General Internal Medicine*, **21**, 320–26.

[18] Misra, A. and Vikram, N.A. (2002) Insulin resistance syndrome (metabolic syndrome) and Asian Indians. *Current Science*, **83**, 1483–96.

[19] Enos, W.F., Holmes, R.H. and Beyer, J. (1953) Coronary disease among United States soldiers killed in action in Korea. *The Journal of the American Medical Association*, **152**, 1090–93.

[20] McNamara, J.J., Molot, M.A., Stremple, J.F. and Cutting, R.T. (1971) Coronary artery disease in combat casualties in Vietnam. *The Journal of the American Medical Association*, **216**, 1185–87.

[21] Joseph, A., Ackerman, D., Talley, J.D. *et al.* (1993) Manifestations of coronary atherosclerosis in young trauma victims – an autopsy study. *Journal of the American College of Cardiology*, **22**, 459–67.

[22] Berenson, G. and Srnivasan, S. (2005) Cardiovascular risk factors in youth with implications for aging: The Bogalusa Heart Study. *Neurobiology of Aging*, **26**, 303–7.

[23] National Cholesterol Education Program Expert Panel on Blood Cholesterol Levels in Children and Adolescents. National Cholesterol Education Program (NCEP) (1992) Highlights of the report of the expert panel on blood cholesterol levels in children and adolescents. *Pediatrics*, **89**, 495–501.

[24] McCrindle, B.W., Urbina, E.M., Dennison, B.A. *et al.* American Heart Association Writing Group (2007) Summary of the American Heart Association's scientific statement on drug therapy of high-risk lipid abnormalities in children and adolescents. *Arteriosclerosis, Thrombosis, and Vascular Biology*, **27**, 982–85.

[25] Daniels, S.R. (2007) Management of dyslipidemia in Children, in *Therapeutic Lipidology*, (eds M.H. Davidson, P.P. Toth and K.C. Maki), Humana Press, Totowa.

9 Emerging Risk Factors and Biomarkers of Cardiovascular Disease

Key Points

- *The use of nontraditional biomarkers to identify coronary heart disease (CHD) risk represents a strategy that may help to better discriminate among individuals that are potential candidates for aggressive risk factor management, and to more effectively treat patients with, or at risk of, CHD.*

- *Ongoing research on the use of biomarkers for CHD risk is helping to define population subgroups who will be most likely to benefit, cost effectively, from measurement and/or treatment of nontraditional risk markers.*

- *At the present time, high-sensitivity C-reactive protein (hsCRP) is the most intensively studied and most valuable biomarker to supplement traditional risk factor evaluation.*

Nearly 80 million US adults have cardiovascular disease (CVD) and it is estimated that at least 90% of patients with CHD have prior exposure to at least one of several major risk factors including high cholesterol, hypertension, diabetes, and cigarette use [1]. Despite much progress in identifying and managing all forms of CVD, CHD remains the leading cause of morbidity and mortality in the USA. While major risk factors such as low-density lipoprotein cholesterol (LDL-C), hypertension, diabetes, and cigarette use are well established in contributing to the development and progression of CHD, several "novel" risk factors are being intensively explored in an effort to further refine our understanding of atherogenesis. This chapter provides an overview of emerging risk factors and biomarkers for CHD including C-reactive protein (CRP), myeloperoxidase, lipoprotein-associated phospholipase A_2, lipoprotein(a), homocysteine, and low-density lipoprotein (LDL) particle number, quantitated by nuclear magnetic resonance (NMR). Each of these molecular species provides additional information about risk for CHD events in both primary and secondary prevention.

9.1   ROLE OF INFLAMMATION IN THE PATHOGENESIS OF ATHEROSCLEROSIS

It is well established that inflammation plays a significant role in the etiology of atherosclerosis (see also Chapter 2 and references therein). Every phase of atherogenesis is significantly influenced by mediators of inflammation [2]. The attraction and accumulation of macrophages, mast cells and activated T cells, the transformation of monocytes into macrophages, and the uptake of modified lipoproteins by macrophages initiate formation of the fatty streak [3]. A large variety of molecules participate in the development of a proinflammatory milieu characteristic of atherosclerosis, including: oxidized LDLs; cytokines such as interleukin-1 and tumor necrosis factor-α; endothelial adhesion molecules (intercellular adhesion molecule 1 (ICAM-1), vascular cell adhesion molecule 1 (VCAM-1)), selectins P and L); and acute phase reactants such as CRP [2]. Quantifying many of these mediators of inflammation can provide a unique vantage point from which to assess a patient's risk for CVD and identify novel targets for therapeutic intervention [4].

9.2   BIOMARKERS OF CARDIOVASCULAR DISEASE

The term biomarker, or biological marker, identifies a quantifiable biological parameter that serves as an index for disease risk or a biological trait [5]. Biomarkers represent alterations in the constituents of tissues or body fluids in response to a stimulus and may be measured in a biological specimen such as serum, or obtained with an imaging test [5]. A number of biomarkers have been identified for quantifying an individual's risk of CVD. The spectrum of biomarkers for identifying patients at risk include those associated with structural and functional arterial vulnerability, blood vulnerability, and myocardial vulnerability measures (Table 9.1). Several prominent biomarkers of arterial vulnerability include inflammatory mediators such as CRP and myeloperoxidase; serological biomarkers including lipoprotein-associated phospholipase A_2, lipoprotein a [Lp(a)], LDL particle number, and homocysteine.

Table 9.1 Biomarkers for identifying cardiovascular disease risk.

- Arterial Vulnerability
  - Serological biomarkers of arterial vulnerability
    - ○ Abnormal lipid profile

      Apolipoprotein B
      Cholesterol ester transfer protein
      Lipoprotein(a)
      Lipoprotein-associated phospholipase A_2

    - ○ Inflammation

      High-sensitivity C-reactive protein
      Interleukin 6
      Interleukin 18
      Serum amyloid A
      Myeloperoxidase
      Soluble intercellular adhesion molecule

    - ○ Homocysteine
    - ○ Oxidized low density lipoprotein
    - ○ Natriuretic peptides
    - ○ Matrix metalloproteinase-9
    - ○ Tissue inhibitor of matrix metallopreteinases-1
  - Structural markers of arterial vulnerability
    - ○ Carotid intimal-medial thickness
    - ○ Coronary artery calcium
  - Functional markers of arterial vulnerability
    - ○ Blood pressure
    - ○ Endothelial dysfunction
    - ○ Arterial stiffness
    - ○ Ankle-brachial index
- Blood vulnerability
  - Serological markers of blood vulnerability
    - ○ Hypercoagulability

      Fibrinogen
      D-dimer

    - ○ Decreased fibrinolysis

      Tissue Plasminogen activator/Plasminogen activator inhibitor-1

    - ○ Increased coagulation factors

      von Willebrand Factor

(continued overleaf)

Table 9.1   *(continued)*

- Myocardial vulnerability
  - Structural markers of myocardial vulnerability
    - ○ Left ventricular hypertrophy
    - ○ Left ventricular dysfunction
  - Functional markers of myocardial vulnerability
    - ○ Exercise stress test/stress echo
    - ○ Positron emission tomography
  - Serological markers of myocardial vulnerability
    - ○ Troponins

Adapted from Vasan, R.S. (2006) Biomarkers of cardiovascular disease: molecular basis and practical considerations. *Circulation*, **113**, 2335–62, [5] with permission from Lippincott Williams & Wilkins.

C-REACTIVE PROTEIN

CRP is an acute phase plasma protein produced by the liver in response to increased systemic expression of interleukin-6. CRP levels rise during inflammation and CRP is thought to assist in the binding of complement to foreign and damaged cells to enhance phagocytosis by macrophages. CRP is an annular, pentameric disc in shape and is a member of the pentraxin family of proteins [6]. Research has established that patients with elevated basal levels of CRP are at an increased risk for CVD [7–9].

Basic scientific research has shown that CRP may contribute to atherogenesis by several mechanisms, including reducing endothelial nitric oxide production, decreasing fibrinolytic capacity and increasing endothelin-1 production, promoting monocyte chemoattractant-1 expression, oxidation of LDL particles, stimulating macrophage scavenging receptor expression, and augmenting complement fixation, among other effects [10–15]. (Figure 9.1).

MEASUREMENT OF CRP

CRP is used to assess the severity of systemic inflammation. While sometimes used interchangeably, hsCRP differs from CRP; hsCRP measures CRP in the range from 0.5 to 10 mg l^{-1}. CRP itself is used to assess the presence of bacterial or viral infection or the presence of inflammatory diseases (such as rheumatoid arthritis and connective tissue disease), and measures CRP in the range from 10 to 1000 mg l^{-1}. Immunoassay laboratory measurement of CRP has a detection limit of 3–5 mg l^{-1}, which although adequate for the clinical utility of CRP in monitoring infection, is not useful in assessing

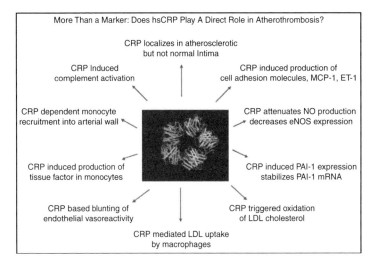

More Than a Marker: Does hsCRP Play A Direct Role in Atherothrombosis?

CRP localizes in atherosclerotic
but not normal Intima

CRP Induced
complement activation

CRP induced production of
cell adhesion molecules, MCP-1, ET-1

CRP dependent monocyte
recruitment into arterial wall

CRP attenuates NO production
decreases eNOS expression

CRP induced production of
tissue factor in monocytes

CRP induced PAI-1 expression
stabilizes PAI-1 mRNA

CRP based blunting of
endothelial vasoreactivity

CRP triggered oxidation
of LDL cholesterol

CRP mediated LDL uptake
by macrophages

Figure 9.1 Role of high-sensitivity C-reactive protein (hsCRP) in atherosclerosis. CRP, C-reactive protein; NO, nitric oxide; eNOS, endothelial nitric oxide synthase; ET-1, endothelin-1; LDL, low-density lipoprotein; MCP-1, monocyte chemoattractant protein-1; PAI-1, plasminogen activator inhibitor-1. Reprinted with permission from Torres, J.L. and Ridker, P.M. (2003) Clinical use of high sensitivity C-reactive protein for the prediction of adverse cardiovascular events. *Current Opinion in Cardiology*, **18**, 471–78, [11] with permission from Lippincott Williams & Wilkins.

and predicting risk of CHD [16]. In contrast, hsCRP is an ultrasensitive assay capable of measuring hsCRP at a concentration of 0.007 mg l^{-1} [16].

hsCRP AS A RISK FACTOR/BIOMARKER FOR CVD EVENTS

A number of prospective epidemiological studies have demonstrated that the plasma level of hsCRP is a strong, independent predictor of risk of future myocardial infarction (MI), stroke, peripheral arterial disease, and vascular death [17–27]. These data are robust and consistent across many prospective studies performed since the mid-1990s. Of considerable importance are the observations that serum levels of hsCRP have been associated with increased vascular event rates among patients with acute coronary ischemia [28–31], stable angina pectoris [32], stable coronary artery disease [33], and a history of MI [34]. In a study of 27 939 healthy women who were followed for MI, stroke, coronary revascularization, or CVD, baseline levels of hsCRP levels were predictive of cardiovascular risk with levels increasing linearly from the very lowest to the very highest levels [9]. Among women with the metabolic syndrome, baseline hsCRP >3.0 portends significantly poorer outcomes than levels <3.0 [35].

hsCRP AS A TARGET OF THERAPY FOR CHD

The clinical relevance of hsCRP in assessing the success of therapy for CHD has been evaluated in several clinical trials. In the Aggrastat-to-Zocor (A to Z) trial comparing early intensive statin treatment (simvastatin 40 mg day^{-1} for 30 days followed by 80 mg day^{-1}) to a delayed conservative statin strategy (placebo for four months followed by 20 mg day^{-1} simvastatin), the prognostic value of hsCRP was assessed during follow-up of 3813 patients with acute coronary syndromes [36]. Serum concentrations of hsCRP were measured at 30 days and four months. Patients with hsCRP >3 mg l^{-1} at 30 days had significantly higher two-year mortality rates compared with those with hsCRP 1–3 mg l^{-1} or <1 mg l^{-1} (6.1% vs 3.7% vs 1.6%, $P <$ 0.0001). Similar results were found with hsCRP measured at four months with hsCRP again showing a significant independent association with all causes of mortality and major cardiovascular events including cardiovascular death, MI, rehospitalization for acute coronary syndrome, or stroke [36]. The cumulative incidence of death from any cause through two years of follow-up was significantly higher in patients with elevated levels of hsCRP >3 mg l^{-1}. Notably, patients receiving intensive statin therapy were more likely to achieve hsCRP levels <1 mg l^{-1} at 30 days ($P = 0.028$) and four months ($P < 0.0001$) compared with patients who received delayed, conservative statin therapy [36].

In addition to being a marker of risk for cardiovascular events, some studies also suggest hsCRP may be a target for therapy. The Pravastatin or Atorvastatin Evaluation and Infection Therapy-Thrombolysis in Myocardial Infarction (PROVE-IT-TIMI) trial investigated the effects of intensive (atorvastatin 80 mg). versus standard (pravastatin 40 mg) daily statin therapy in the prevention of recurrent coronary events among 4162 patients with acute coronary syndromes. The results demonstrated that those patients achieving LDL-C <70 mg dl^{-1} and hsCRP <2 mg l^{-1} had the lowest risk of a recurrent heart attack or coronary death compared with patients who did not achieve these thresholds [37]. (Figure 9.2) These results were consistent with those from the A to Z trial. (Figure 9.2) The Reversal of Atherosclerosis with Aggressive Lipid Lowering (REVERSAL), intensive lipid-lowering (atorvastatin 80 mg) compared with moderate lipid-lowering (pravastatin 40 mg) in 654 patients with stable CHD demonstrated that the rate of progression of coronary artery atheroma volume was significantly and independently associated with the magnitude of reduction in hsCRP during the course of the trial [38]. Patients with CHD who still have CRP levels >2.0 will likely benefit from intensification of both their statin

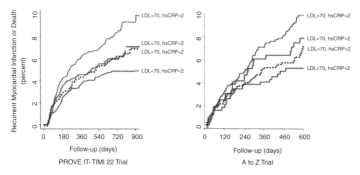

Figure 9.2 Low-density lipoprotein (LDL) cholesterol, high-sensitivity C-reactive protein (hsCRP) and clinical outcomes on statin therapy. Cumulative rates of recurrent myocardial infarction or cardiovascular death among statin-treated patients according to achieved levels of LDL cholesterol in mg dl^{-1} and achieved levels of hsCRP in mg l^{-1} in the PROVE-IT–TIMI-22 (Pravastatin or Atorvastatin Evaluation and Infection Therapy–Thrombolysis in Myocardial Infarction-22) trial **(left)** and in the A to Z (Aggrastat to Zocor) trial **(right)**. Reprinted with permission from Ridker, P.M. (2007) C-reactive protein and the prediction of cardiovascular events among those at intermediate risk: moving an inflammatory hypothesis toward consensus. *Journal of the American College of Cardiology*, **49**, 2129–38, [39]. A full-color version of this figure appears in the color plate section of this book.

therapy and lifestyle modification (weight loss, smoking cessation, dietary modification), which have demonstrated efficacy for lowering the hsCRP concentration. However, direct evidence from clinical trials to prospectively test this hypothesis is not yet available.

AHA/CDC RECOMMENDATIONS ON USE OF hsCRP FOR STRATIFYING CHD RISK

Various CHD risk factors, metabolic syndrome, and diabetes mellitus are strongly associated with serum levels of hsCRP [7, 19, 40, 41]. The Centers for Disease Control and Prevention and the American Heart Association issued clinical guidelines for CRP measurement and define serum hsCRP levels of <1, 1 to <3 and ≥3 mg l^{-1} as consistent with low, moderate, and high risk for CVD [2, 33]. The CDC/AHA guidelines recommended that hsCRP measurements be targeted toward patients with a Framingham risk score that places them at moderate to moderately high risk. Patients at low or high risk are not currently advised to undergo screening for hsCRP [11]. Patients at moderate risk who have an hsCRP >3.0 should be treated as being at high risk for CHD.

MYELOPEROXIDASE

Myeloperoxidase is a heme protein secreted by activated macrophages and is recognized as a potentiator of atherosclerosis [42]. Myeloperoxidase is a pro-oxidative enzyme used by macrophages and neutrophils to inactivate bacteria during infection. As part of its function in innate host defense, myeloperoxidase generates reactive oxidant species that can subsequently contribute to inflammatory injury [43]. It has been identified as a catalyst for the generation of numerous reactive oxidants and diffusible radical species that are capable of promoting lipoprotein oxidation [42, 44, 45]. The identification of the expression of myeloperoxidase in atherosclerotic plaque [46] and the demonstration of the links between myeloperoxidase and oxidative damage to proteins and lipids [47–49] has implicated the enzyme as a participant in atherogenesis.

In addition to its role in generating atherogenic lipoproteins, myeloperoxidase promotes atherogenesis by: (i) generating oxygen free radicals that can interact with nitric oxide thereby forming peroxynitrite radicals which can induce protein nitration and lipid peroxidation; (ii) inducing endothelial dysfunction and leukocyte transmigration; (iii) foam cell formation; and (iv) activation of metalloproteinase and cellular apoptosis, leading to weakening and breakdown of the fibrous cap overlying atheromatous plaques (Table 9.2) [42, 50, 51]. Consequently, myeloperoxidase, like hsCRP, is not only a marker of CHD risk, but is also intimately involved in some of the most important mechanisms driving atherogenesis.

Myeloperoxidase has been found to selectively bind to apolipoprotein A-I [52]. *In vitro* studies have demonstrated that myeloperoxidase-generated oxidants, including hypochlorus acid, may interfere with the normal interaction of apolipoprotein A-I with scavenger receptor B1, impairing high-density lipoprotein (HDL)-dependent selective lipid efflux and reverse cholesterol transport [53]. While myeloperoxidase is acknowledged to be a marker of risk for MI, stroke, and coronary death, there is uncertainty as how best to develop targeted therapeutic interventions to inhibit its action due to potential adverse effects related to impairment in the role of enzymes in innate host defenses [42]. Currently, there are no national guidelines outlining the appropriate use of myeloperoxidase, but continued research may shed further light on its role in screening and elucidate the full scope of its activity in regulating atherogenesis.

LIPOPROTEIN-ASSOCIATED PHOSPHOLIPASE A_2

Lipoprotein-associated phospholipase A_2 (Lp-PLA$_2$) has recently emerged as an independent inflammatory marker of CVD risk. Lp-PLA$_2$, also known as *platelet activating factor acetylhydrolase* (PAF-AH), is a member of the phospholipase A_2 family of enzymes [54, 55]. It is a calcium-independent serine lipase that is produced predominantly by macrophages and circulates

Table 9.2 The role of myeloperoxidase in cardiovascular disease.

- Plaque initiation and progression
  - Lipid peroxidation
  - Catalytic consumption of nitric oxide
  - Formation of bioactive lipids
  - Leukocyte chemotaxis

- Generation of atherogenic low-density lipoprotein
  - Generation of dysfunctional high-density lipoprotein

- Plaque Vulnerability
  - Tissue factor activation

- Protease activation
  - Endothelial cell apoptosis

- Myocardial Injury
  - Protease activation
  - Degradation of extracellular matrix

- Adverse ventricular remodeling

- Heart failure

Adapted from Nicholls, S.J. and Hazen, S.L. (2005) Myeloperoxidase and cardiovascular disease. *Arteriosclerosis, Thrombosis and Vascular Biology*, **25**, 1102–111, [42] with kind permission of Lippincott Williams & Wilkins.

bound mainly to the Apo B-100 moiety of LDL [56]. Epidemiologic studies have demonstrated a strong independent association between elevated levels of Lp-PLA$_2$ and risk of CHD events, including non-fatal MI, death from CHD, need for revascularization procedures, and ischemic stroke [55, 57–62]. (Table 9.3 and Figure 9.3).

The molecular basis for the relationship between Lp-PLA$_2$ and the development of atherosclerosis is complex. Lp-PLA$_2$ hydrolyzes phospholipids, which leads to the modulation of lipoprotein particle phospholipid content and size, as well as the production of proinflammatory intermediates [64–66]. Lp-PLA$_2$ hydrolyzes oxidized phospholipids to generate lysophosphatidylcholine and oxidized fatty acids, both of which promote inflammation [67]. Lp-PLA$_2$ may play a direct role in the development of endothelial dysfunction [68, 69] as lysophosphatidylcholine has been demonstrated to: (i) upregulate the expression of adhesion molecules, cytokines, and CD40 ligand; (ii) stimulate macrophage proliferation, neutrophil activation, T cell production of cytokines, and migration of smooth muscle cells; (iii) inhibit endothelium-derived nitric oxide production; and (iv) increase monocyte

Table 9.3 Plasma levels of lipoprotein-associated phospholipase A_2 (Lp-PLA$_2$) and the risk of cardiovascular events in primary prevention populations.

Study	Design	Cases/non-cases	End point	Follow-up (y)	Lp-PLA$_2$ assay	Lp-PLA$_2$ cases vs non-cases	Adjusted HR (95% CI)
WOSCOPS[e]	Nested case-control	580/1160	CHD death, MI, revascularization	5	Mass	Higher	1.18 (1.05–1.33; $P = 0.005$)[a]
WHS[f]	Nested case-control	123/123	CHD death, MI, stroke	3	Mass	Higher	1.17 (0.45–3.05; NS)[b]
ARIC[g,h]	Case cohort	608/740	CHD death, MI, revascularization	6	Mass	Higher	1.15 (0.81–1.63; NS)[c] 2.08 (1.20–3.62; $P < 0.05$)[c,d]
		194/766	Ischemic stroke	6	Mass	Higher	1.93 (1.14–3.27; $P = 0.015$)[c]
MONICA[i]	Cohort	97/837	CHD death, MI	14	Mass	Higher	1.21 (1.01–1.45; $P = 0.04$)[a]
Rotterdam[j]	Case cohort	308/1822	CHD death, MI	7	Activity	Higher	1.96 (1.25–3.09; $P = 0.02$)[c]
		110/1822	Ischemic stroke	6	Activity	Higher	1.95 (1.02–3.73; $P = 0.04$)[c]

[a]Increase of 1 SD.
[b]With the lowest quartile as the reference.
[c]With the lowest tertile as the reference.
[d]In population with baseline LDL <130 mg dl^{-1}.
ARIC, Atherosclerosis Risk In Communities study; CHD, coronary heart disease; CRP, C-reactive protein; HR, hazard ratio adjusted for age, smoking, diabetes mellitus, gender, systolic blood pressure, LDL cholesterol (or total cholesterol/HDL or non-HDL cholesterol), high-sensitivity CRP, and other variables; MI, myocardial infarction; MONICA, the MONItoring of trends and determinants in CArdiovascular disease in men in Augsburg survey; WHS, the Women's Health Study; WOSCOPS, the West Of Scotland Coronary Prevention Study.

[e]Packard, C.J., O'Reilly, D.S., Caslake, M.J. et al. (2000) Lipoprotein-associated phospholipase A_2 as an independent predictor of coronary heart disease. West of Scotland Coronary Prevention Study Group. The New England Journal of Medicine, **343**, 1148–55, [55].

[f]Blake, G.J., Dada, N., Fox, J.C. et al. (2001) A prospective evaluation of lipoprotein-associated phospholipase A(2) levels and the risk of future cardiovascular events in women. Journal of the American College of Cardiology, **38**, 1302–6, [63].

[g]Ballantyne, C.M. Hoogeveen, R.C., Bang, H. et al. (2005) Lipoprotein-associated phospholipase A_2, high-sensitivity C-reactive protein, and risk for incident ischemic stroke in middle-aged men and women in the Atherosclerosis Risk in Communities (ARIC) study. Archives of Internal Medicine, **165**, 2479–84, [57].

[h]Ballantyne, C.M. Hoogeveen, R.C., Bang, H. et al. (2004) Lipoprotein-associated phospholipase A_2, high-sensitivity C-reactive protein, and risk for incident coronary heart disease in middle-aged men and women in the Atherosclerosis Risk in Communities (ARIC) study. Circulation, **109**, 837–42, [58].

[i]Koenig, W., Khuseyinova, N., Lowel, H. et al. (2004) Lipoprotein-associated phospholipase A_2 adds to risk prediction of incident coronary events by C-reactive protein in apparently healthy middle-aged men from the general population: results from the 14-year follow-up of a large cohort from southern Germany. Circulation, **110**, 1903–8, [62].

[j]Oei, H.H., van der Meer, I.M., Hofman, A. et al. (2005) Lipoprotein-associated phospholipase A_2 activity is associated with risk of coronary heart disease and ischemic stroke: the Rotterdam Study. Circulation, **111**, 570–75, [61].

Reproduced with permission from Zalewski, A. and Macphee, C. (2005) Role of lipoprotein-associated phospholipase A_2 in atherosclerosis: biology, epidemiology, and possible therapeutic target. Arteriosclerosis, Thrombosis and Vascular Biology, **25**, 923–31 with kind permission of Lippincott Williams & Wilkins.

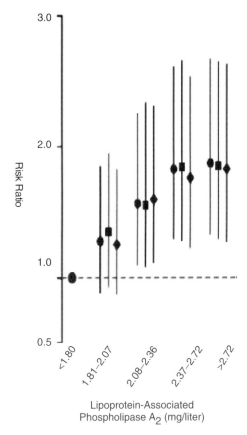

Figure 9.3   Lipoprotein-associated phospholipase A_2 as an independent predictor of coronary heart disease. Relationship of lipoprotein-associated phospholipase A_2 to coronary events (non-fatal myocardial infarction, death from coronary heart disease, or need for revascularization procedure) in 580 men. Vertical bars denote 95% confidence intervals; circles indicate unadjusted relative risks, squares indicate relative risks adjusted for C-reactive protein levels, white-cell count and fibrinogen levels; diamonds indicate risk ratios adjusted for age, systolic blood pressure, plasma triglyceride levels, low-density lipoprotein cholesterol levels, and high-density lipoprotein cholesterol levels. Reproduced with permission from Packard, C.J., O'Reilly, D.S., Caslake, M.J. *et al.* (2000) Lipoprotein-associated phospholipase A_2 as an independent predictor of coronary heart disease. West of Scotland Coronary Prevention Study Group. *New England Journal of Medicine*, **343**, 1148–55, [55].

chemoattractant protein-1 (MCP-1) expression, thereby promoting monocyte uptake into the subendothelial space [70, 71].

The expression of Lp-PLA$_2$ has been demonstrated within coronary atheromas and it is expressed by macrophages within the fibrous cap region of rupture-prone and ruptured lesions [72]. Of interest is that elevated levels of Lp-PLA$_2$ have not been found to correlate with the elevation of other inflammatory markers including hsCRP, interleukin-6, or white blood cell count, suggesting this enzyme has an independent role in atherogenesis [56]. Several commercial assays are available for Lp-PLA$_2$ testing; however, uniform reporting of cut points or decision values for classifying risk have not been established [71]. There are currently no guidelines or recommendations for the use of Lp-PLA$_2$ in clinical practice. It has been proposed that the measurement of Lp-PLA$_2$ be used in intermediate-risk persons to determine the need for reclassification to a higher cardiovascular risk category [71].

LIPOPROTEIN(a)

Lipoprotein(a) [Lp(a)] is a lipoprotein subclass that has been identified as a major risk factor for CVD. Lp(a) is a member of the LDL class of lipoproteins and is structurally similar to LDL in both protein and lipid composition, but is different due to the presence of the unique glycoprotein moiety called *apolipoprotein(a)* [*apo (a)*] [73, 74]. Lp(a) was first discovered by Berg in 1963 [75] and since that time numerous studies have established that high plasma Lp(a) concentrations are associated with a variety of cardiovascular disorders including CHD, peripheral vascular disease, ischemic stroke, and abdominal aortic aneurysm [74, 76].

Lp(a) is considered to have both proatherogenic properties because of its similarity to LDL, as well as prothrombotic properties due to the similarity of apo(a) to plasminogen [74]. (Figure 9.4). Studies have demonstrated that Lp(a) accumulates in the arterial wall at the sites of human atherosclerotic lesions [77] and in coronary atheroma specimens [78]. The exact role of Lp(a) in atherogenesis is not well understood, but it has been demonstrated to be an independent risk factor through many studies including a meta-analysis of 27 prospective cohorts involving 5436 patients [79].

While normal values of Lp(a) are below 30 mg dl^{-1}, ethnic differences have been demonstrated [80], and levels appear to be genetically influenced, mostly by a well-characterized size polymorphism in the apo(a) gene [81]. A significant issue in the use of Lp(a) values in the clinical setting is the discrepancy in the values generated by different measurement methods, which makes it difficult to compare results from different studies [73]. The defined threshold of Lp(a) concentration at which individuals can be classified as being at increased risk for CHD varies among studies,

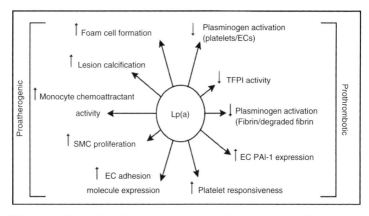

Figure 9.4 Potential pathogenic mechanisms of lipoprotein(a). Lipoprotein(a) [Lp(a)] has proatherogenic properties because it is a type of LDL and prothrombotic properties due to the similarity of apoprotein(a) to plasminogen. This diagram outlines the effects of Lp(a) that have been demonstrated by *in vitro* studies or in animal models of apo(a)/Lp(a). Mechanisms that are proatherogenic are shown to the left while those that are potentially prothrombotic are shown to the right. To date, none of these mechanisms have been directly demonstrated to be mediated by Lp(a) in human disease. EC, endothelial cell; SMC, smooth muscle cell; PAI-1, plasminogen activator inhibitor-1; TFPI, tissue factor pathway inhibitor. Reprinted with permission from Marcovina, S.M. and Koschinsky, M.L. (2003) Evaluation of lipoprotein(a) as a prothrombotic factor: progress from bench to bedside. *Current Opinion in Lipidology*, **14**, 361–66, [74].

ranging from Lp(a) values of 20–40 mg dl^{-1} [73]. These differences can hamper clinical interpretation of values and lead to erroneous assignment of cardiovascular risk category.

Currently, there are no national guidelines outlining recommendations for screening of Lp(a). Additionally, there is no prospective clinical trial evidence that treating Lp(a) is associated with reduced risk for cardiovascular events. The lack of evidence of a causal role of Lp(a) in human CHD as well as lack of understanding of the definitive mechanisms underlying the pathophysiology of Lp(a) has hindered the development of therapies specifically designed to lower plasma Lp(a) levels [73]. Unlike other plasma lipoproteins, Lp(a) is not substantially impacted by diet or most lipid-lowering drugs [74]. Niacin, alone and in combination with statin therapy, has been demonstrated to lower Lp(a) levels, but only modestly (approximately 20–25% at maximal doses of niacin) [82–84]. There is no clinical trial evidence that this approach to Lp(a) lowering impacts cardiovascular outcomes. Lp(a) apheresis procedures have demonstrated a capacity to decrease Lp(a) concentrations by 50% or more, yet the technique is expensive and reserved for extreme cases of heterozygous and homozygous familial hyperlipidemia [73]. Screening of the general population for Lp(a) is not recommended and there are no national guidelines on its treatment, nor has a treatment target been specified. However, consistent with a National Heart, Lung, and Blood Institute conference on Lp(a), measurement of Lp(a) can be considered in patients with a history of CHD and a "normal" lipid profile, or patients with a strong family history for premature CHD [85]. In these patients, it becomes especially important to treat lipids to NCEP target levels and to make sure other risk factors are identified and rigorously controlled to national guideline levels.

HOMOCYSTEINE

Homocysteine is an amino acid produced from the metabolism of methionine [86]. Epidemiological investigations have demonstrated that elevated serum homocysteine is related to risk of CHD, cerebrovascular accident, and peripheral vascular disease. Hyperhomocysteinemia is also associated with hypercoagulability and increased risk for deep venous thrombosis and pulmonary embolism. The proposed mechanisms of adverse vascular effects of homocysteine include endothelial injury from increased production of peroxides and reduced glutathione peroxidase activity; reduced nitric oxide availability and increased vessel vasoconstriction, increased platelet activation and aggregation, and dysregulation of the coagulation system secondary to increased production of tissue factor; depressed activity of protein C; and reduced expression of thrombomodulin and tissue plasminogen activator activity [87]. Hyperhomocysteinemia is also associated with impaired hepatic capacity to produce Apo A-I and HDL [88].

Reference ranges for homocysteine are calculated as 95% reference ranges (mean ± 2 standard deviations) using the distribution of values obtained for healthy individuals. Therefore, an elevated blood level of homocysteine (hyperhomocysteinemia) is established if the total serum homocysteine concentration is more than 2 standard deviations above the mean [89]. Normal total plasma homocysteine levels range from 5 to 15 μmol l^{-1}, with hyperhomocysteinemia being classified as mild at levels of 15–30 μmol l^{-1}, intermediate between 31 and 100 μmol l^{-1}, and severe at >100 μmol l^{-1} [90, 91]. Elevated homocysteine levels can be caused by several factors, including folate and vitamin B$_6$ and B$_{12}$ deficiency, diabetes mellitus, and various drugs such as fenofibrate [92]. Other common causes of elevated homocysteine levels include genetic defects and renal insufficiency/failure [89]. Several enzyme deficiencies are associated with hyperhomocysteinemia including thiolase, cystathionine beta-synthase, and methylenetetrahydrofolate reductase. Numerous mutations in these enzymes have been characterized.

Clinical trial data supports an association between elevated homocysteine levels and increased risk of CHD [93]. However, whether lowering homocysteine levels by administration of folate with or without vitamins B_6 and B_{12} is associated with any significant decrease in vascular risk remains controversial as no beneficial impact on cardiovascular risk has been demonstrated in several large clinical trials [92, 94–97]. Although fluorescence polarization immunoassay has greatly improved the measurement of homocysteine, standardized methods are not yet available. Currently, there are no specific recommendations by either primary care or specialty societies for screening patients for elevated homocysteine levels. In addition, there is no consensus as to the optimal dose of folic acid and other B vitamins to use for the treatment of elevated blood homocysteine levels. To simply assume that the use of folate with vitamins B_6 and B_{12} is benign is premature. In one study of folate supplementation in patients undergoing percutaneous coronary luminal angioplasty with stent placement, patients receiving folate therapy experienced higher rates of in-stent restenosis compared with the placebo group [98]. However, ongoing research on the role of folic acid therapy in patients with hyperhomocysteinemia may provide additional information on the benefits of targeting treatment for the primary prevention of CHD and the secondary prevention of cardiovascular events. The Study of the Effectiveness of Additional Reductions in Cholesterol and Homocysteine (SEARCH) trial is underway and should lend important additional information to this issue [99].

LDL PARTICLE NUMBER QUANTITATED BY NMR

LDL particles are involved in the pathogenesis of atherosclerotic disease and quantitative analysis of LDL particles can be useful in determining CHD risk. LDL particles vary in size and density, and studies have identified that a pattern that has more small dense LDL particles (pattern B) is associated with higher CHD risk compared with larger size LDL (pattern A) [100]. NMR provides a spectroscopic means of quantifying LDL particles and of measuring LDL particle size. As a normal LDL-C can be associated with very high serum levels of LDL particles and excess risk for CHD, the quantitation of LDL particle number confers additional information not gleaned from LDL-C.

However, the risk for atherosclerosis has been demonstrated to be related more to particle number, rather than particle size. All sizes of LDL are atherogenic. LDL particle number measured by NMR has been shown to be a strong, independent predictor of CHD. Importantly, LDL particle number is a strong predictor for the development of CHD in women [101, 102], as well as a predictor of the rate of CVD progression [103].

While NMR lipoprotein analysis is theoretically appealing as it allows quantitative assessment of lipoproteins, there are currently no established recommendations for routine use of NMR lipoprotein analysis. Future re-breaksearch may identify subsets of individuals whose risk is underestimated by conventional lipid analysis and who may benefit from NMR lipoprotein analysis [100].

REFERENCES

[1] Association AH (2007) *Heart Disease and Stroke Statistics – 2007 Update*, American Heart Association, Dallas.

[2] Pearson T.A., Mensah G.A., Alexander R.W. *et al.* (2003) Markers of inflammation and cardiovascular disease: application to clinical and public health practice: a statement for healthcare professionals from the Centers for Disease Control and Prevention and the American Heart Association. *Circulation*, **107**, 499–511.

[3] Libby, P. (2002) Inflammation in atherosclerosis. *Nature*, **420**, 868–74.

[4] Tsimikas, S. (2006) Oxidative biomarkers in the diagnosis and prognosis of cardiovascular disease. *The American Journal of Cardiology*, **98**, 4.

[5] Vasan, R.S. (2006) Biomarkers of cardiovascular disease: molecular basis and practical considerations. *Circulation*, **113**, 2335–62.

[6] Ridker, P.M., Bassuk, S.S., Toth, P.P. (2003) C-reactive protein and risk of cardiovascular disease: evidence and clinical application. *Current Atherosclerosis Report*, **5**, 341–49.

[7] Ndumele, C.E., Pradhan, A.D. and Ridker, P.M. (2006) Interrelationships between inflammation, C-reactive protein, and insulin resistance. *Journal of the Cardio Metabolic Syndrome*, **1**, 190–96.

[8] Danesh, J., Wheeler, J.G., Hirschfield, G.M. *et al.* (2004) C-reactive protein and other circulating markers of inflammation in the prediction of coronary heart disease. *The New England Journal of Medicine*, **350**, 1387–97.

[9] Ridker, P.M.C.N. (2004) Clinical usefulness of very high and very low levels of c-reactive protein across the full range of Framingham risk scores. *Circulation*, **109**, 1955–59.

[10] Devaraj, S., Xu, D.Y. and Jialal, I. (2003) C-reactive protein increases plasminogen activator inhibitor-1 expression and activity in human aortic endothelial cells: implications for the metabolic syndrome and atherothrombosis. *Circulation*, **107**, 398–404.

[11] Torres, J.L. and Ridker, P.M. (2003) Clinical use of high sensitivity C-reactive protein for the prediction of adverse cardiovascular events. *Current Opinion in Cardiology*, **18**, 471–78.

[12] Venugopal, S.K., Devaraj, S., Yuhanna, I. *et al.* (2002) Demonstration that C-reactive protein decreases eNOS expression and bioactivity in human aortic endothelial cells. *Circulation*, **106**, 1439–41.

[13] Verma, S., Wang, C.H., Li, S.H. *et al.* (2002) A self-fulfilling prophecy: C-reactive protein attenuates nitric oxide production and inhibits angiogenesis. *Circulation*, **106**, 913–19.

[14] Fichtlscherer, S., Rosenberger, G., Walter, D.H. *et al.* (2000) Elevated C-reactive protein levels and impaired endothelial vasoreactivity in patients with coronary artery disease. *Circulation*, **102**, 1000–6.

[15] Ridker, P.M., Bassuk, S.S. and Toth, P.P. (2003) C-reactive protein and risk of cardiovascular disease: evidence and clinical application. *Current Atherosclerosis Report*, **5**, 341–49.

[16] Rifai, N., Tracy, R.P. and Ridker, P.M. (1999) Clinical efficacy of an automated high-sensitivity C-reactive protein assay. *Clinical Chemistry*, **45**, 2136–41.

[17] Ridker, P.M., Hennekens, C.H., Buring, J.E. and Rifai, N. (2000) C-reactive protein and other markers of inflammation in the prediction of cardiovascular disease in women. *The New England Journal of Medicine*, **342**, 836–43.

[18] Ridker, P.M., Rifai, N., Pfeffer, M.A. *et al.* (1998) Inflammation, pravastatin, and the risk of coronary events after myocardial infarction in patients with average cholesterol levels. Cholesterol and Recurrent Events (CARE) Investigators. *Circulation*, **98**, 839–44.

[19] Ridker, P.M., Cushman, M., Stampfer, M.J. *et al.* (1998) Plasma concentration of C-reactive protein and risk of developing peripheral vascular disease. *Circulation*, **97**, 425–28.

[20] Ridker, P.M., Cushman, M., Stampfer, M.J. *et al.* (1997) Inflammation, aspirin, and the risk of cardiovascular disease in apparently healthy men. [erratum appears in (1997) The New England Journal of Medicine, 337(5), 356]. *The New England Journal of Medicine*, **336**, 973–9.

[21] Koenig, W., Sund, M., Frohlich, M. *et al.* (1999) C-Reactive protein, a sensitive marker of inflammation, predicts future risk of coronary heart disease in initially healthy middle-aged men: results from the MONICA (Monitoring Trends and Determinants in Cardiovascular Disease) Augsburg Cohort Study, 1984–1992. *Circulation*, **99**, 237–42.

[22] Kuller, L.H., Tracy, R.P., Shaten, J. and Meilahn, E.N. (1996) Relation of C-reactive protein and coronary heart disease in the MRFIT nested case-control study. Multiple Risk Factor Intervention Trial. *American Journal of Epidemiology*, **144**, 537–47.

[23] Tracy, R.P., Lemaitre, R.N., Psaty, B.M. *et al.* (1997) Relationship of C-reactive protein to risk of cardiovascular disease in the elderly. Results from the Cardiovascular Health Study and the Rural Health Promotion Project. *Arteriosclerosis, Thrombosis and Vascular Biology*, **17**, 1121–27.

[24] Roivainen, M., Viik-Kajander, M., Palosuo, T. *et al.* (2000) Infections, inflammation, and the risk of coronary heart disease. *Circulation*, **101**, 252–57.

[25] Harris, T.B., Ferrucci, L., Tracy, R.P. *et al.* (1999) Associations of elevated interleukin-6 and C-reactive protein levels with mortality in the elderly. *The American Journal of Medicine*, **106**, 506–12.

[26] Mendall, M.A., Strachan, D.P., Butland, B.K. *et al.* (2000) C-reactive protein: relation to total mortality, cardiovascular mortality and cardiovascular risk factors in men. *European Heart Journal*, **21**, 1584–90.

[27] Danesh, J., Collins, R. and Peto, R. (2000) Lipoprotein(a) and coronary heart disease. Meta-analysis of prospective studies. *Circulation*, **102**, 1082–85.

[28] Liuzzo, G., Biasucci, L.M., Gallimore, J.R. *et al.* (1994) The prognostic value of C-reactive protein and serum amyloid a protein in severe unstable angina. *The New England Journal of Medicine*, **331**, 417–24.

[29] Morrow, D.A., Rifai, N., Antman, E.M. *et al.* (1998) C-reactive protein is a potent predictor of mortality independently of and in combination with troponin T in acute coronary syndromes: a TIMI 11A substudy. Thrombolysis

in Myocardial Infarction. *Journal of the American College of Cardiology*, **31**, 1460–65.

[30] Biasucci, L.M., Liuzzo, G., Grillo, R.L. *et al.* (1999) Elevated levels of C-reactive protein at discharge in patients with unstable angina predict recurrent instability. *Circulation*, **99**, 855–60.

[31] Toss, H., Lindahl, B., Siegbahn, A. and Wallentin, L. (1997) Prognostic influence of increased fibrinogen and C-reactive protein levels in unstable coronary artery disease. FRISC Study Group. Fragmin during instability in coronary artery disease. *Circulation*, **96**, 4204–10.

[32] Lindahl, B., Toss, H., Siegbahn, A. *et al.* (2000) Markers of myocardial damage and inflammation in relation to long-term mortality in unstable coronary artery disease. FRISC Study Group. Fragmin during Instability in Coronary Artery Disease. *The New England Journal of Medicine*, **343**, 1139–47.

[33] Sabatine, M.S., Morrow, D.A., Jablonski, K.A. *et al.* (2007) Prognostic significance of the centers for disease control/american heart association high-sensitivity C-reactive protein cut points for cardiovascular and other outcomes in patients with stable coronary artery disease. *Circulation*, **115**, 1528–36.

[34] Haverkate, F., Thompson, S.G., Pyke, S.D. *et al.* (1997) Production of C-reactive protein and risk of coronary events in stable and unstable angina. European Concerted Action on Thrombosis and Disabilities Angina Pectoris Study Group. *Lancet*, **349**, 462–66.

[35] Ridker, P.M., Buring, J.E., Cook, N.R. and Rifai, N. (2003) C-reactive protein, the metabolic syndrome, and risk of incident cardiovascular events: an 8-year follow-up of 14 719 initially healthy American women. *Circulation*, **107**, 391–97.

[36] Morrow, D.A., de Lemos, J.A., Sabatine, M.S. *et al.* (2006) Clinical relevance of C-reactive protein during follow-up of patients with acute coronary syndromes in the Aggrastat-to-Zocor Trial. *Circulation*, **114**, 281–88.

[37] Ahmed, S., Cannon, C.P., Murphy, S.A. and Braunwald, E. (2006) Acute coronary syndromes and diabetes: Is intensive lipid lowering beneficial? Results of the PROVE IT-TIMI 22 trial. *European Heart Journal*, **27**, 2323–29.

[38] Nissen, S.E. (2004) Aggressive lipid-lowering therapy and regression of coronary atheroma. *Journal of the American Medical Association*, **292**, 1–3.

[39] Ridker, P.M. (2007) C-reactive protein and the prediction of cardiovascular events among those at intermediate risk: moving an inflammatory hypothesis toward consensus. *Journal of the American College of Cardiology*, **49**, 2129–38.

[40] Ridker, P.M. (2001) High-sensitivity C-reactive protein: potential adjunct for global risk assessment in the primary prevention of cardiovascular disease. *Circulation*, **103**, 1813–18.

[41] Pradhan, A.D., Manson, J.E., Rifai, N. *et al.* (2001) C-reactive protein, interleukin 6, and risk of developing type 2 diabetes mellitus. *Journal of the American Medical Association*, **286**, 327–34.

[42] Nicholls, S.J. and Hazen, S.L. (2005) Myeloperoxidase and cardiovascular disease. *Arteriosclerosis, Thrombosis and Vascular Biology*, **25**, 1102–111.

[43] Brennan, M.L. and Hazen, S.L. (2003) Emerging role of myeloperoxidase and oxidant stress markers in cardiovascular risk assessment. *Current Opinion in Lipidology*, **14**, 353–59.

[44] Zhang, R., Shen, Z., Nauseef, W.M. and Hazen, S.L. (2002) Defects in leukocyte-mediated initiation of lipid peroxidation in plasma as studied in myeloperoxidase-deficient subjects: systematic identification of multiple endogenous diffusible substrates for myeloperoxidase in plasma. *Blood*, **99**, 1802–10.

[45] Zhang, R., Brennan, M.L., Shen, Z. *et al.* (2002) Myeloperoxidase functions as a major enzymatic catalyst for initiation of lipid peroxidation at sites of inflammation. *Journal of Biological Chemistry*, **277**, 46116–122.

[46] Daugherty, A.D.J., Rateri, D.L. and Heinecke, J.W. (1994) Myeloperoxidase, a catalyst for lipoprotein oxidation, is expressed in human atherosclerotic lesions. *Journal of Clinical Investigation*, **94**, 437–44.

[47] Sepe, S.M. and Clark, R.A. (1985) Oxidant membrane injury by the neutrophil myeloperoxidase system. II. Injury by stimulated neutrophils and protection by lipid-soluble antioxidants. *Journal of Immunology*, **134**, 1896–901.

[48] Heinecke, J.W., Li, W., Francis, G.A. and Goldstein, J.A. (1993) Tyrosyl radical generated by myeloperoxidase catalyzes the oxidative cross-linking of proteins. *Journal of Clinical Investigation*, **91**, 2866–72.

[49] Heinecke, J.W., Li, W., Daehnke, H.L. and Goldstein, J.A. 3rd (1993) Dityrosine, a specific marker of oxidation, is synthesized by the myeloperoxidase-hydrogen peroxide system of human neutrophils and macrophages. *Journal of Biological Chemistry*, **268**, 4069–77.

[50] Vita, J.A., Brennan, M.L., Gokce, N. *et al.* (2004) Serum myeloperoxidase levels independently predict endothelial dysfunction in humans. *Circulation*, **110**, 1134–39.

[51] Carr, A.C., McCall, M.R. and Frei, B. (2000) Oxidation of LDL by myeloperoxidase and reactive nitrogen species: reaction pathways and antioxidant protection. *Arteriosclerosis, Thrombosis and Vascular Biology*, **20**, 1716–23.

[52] Zheng, L., Nukuna, B., Brennan, M.L. *et al.* (2004) Apolipoprotein A-I is a selective target for myeloperoxidase-catalyzed oxidation and functional impairment in subjects with cardiovascular disease. *Journal of Clinical Investigation*, **114**, 529–41.

[53] Marsche, G., Hammer, A., Oskolkova, O. *et al.* (2002) Hypochlorite-modified high density lipoprotein, a high affinity ligand to scavenger receptor class B, type I, impairs high density lipoprotein-dependent selective lipid uptake and reverse cholesterol transport. *Journal of Biological Chemistry*, **277**, 32172–79.

[54] Dada, N., Kim, N.W. and Wolfert, R.L. (2002) Lp-PLA2: an emerging biomarker of coronary heart disease. *Expert Review of Molecular Diagnostics*, **2**, 17–22.

[55] Packard, C.J., O'Reilly, D.S., Caslake, M.J. *et al.* (2000) Lipoprotein-associated phospholipase A$_2$ as an independent predictor of coronary heart disease. West of Scotland Coronary Prevention Study Group. *The New England Journal of Medicine*, **343**, 1148–55.

[56] McConnell, J.P. and Hoefner, D.M. (2006) Lipoprotein-associated phospholipase A$_2$. *Clinics in Laboratory Medicine*, **26**, 679–97.

[57] Ballantyne, C.M., Hoogeveen, R.C., Bang, H. *et al.* (2005) Lipoprotein-associated phospholipase A$_2$, high-sensitivity C-reactive protein, and risk

for incident ischemic stroke in middle-aged men and women in the Atherosclerosis Risk in Communities (ARIC) study. *Archives of Internal Medicine*, **165**, 2479–84.

[58] Ballantyne, C.M., Hoogeveen, R.C., Bang, H. *et al.* (2004) Lipoprotein-associated phospholipase A_2, high-sensitivity C-reactive protein, and risk for incident coronary heart disease in middle-aged men and women in the Atherosclerosis Risk in Communities (ARIC) study. *Circulation*, **109**, 837–42.

[59] Khuseyinova, N., Imhof, A., Rothenbacher, D. *et al.* (2005) Association between Lp-PLA2 and coronary artery disease: focus on its relationship with lipoproteins and markers of inflammation and hemostasis. *Atherosclerosis*, **182**, 181–88.

[60] Brilakis, E.S., McConnell, J.P., Lennon, R.J. *et al.* (2005) Association of lipoprotein-associated phospholipase A_2 levels with coronary artery disease risk factors, angiographic coronary artery disease, and major adverse events at follow-up. *European Heart Journal*, **26**, 137–44.

[61] Oei, H.H., van der Meer, I.M., Hofman, A. *et al.* (2005) Lipoprotein-associated phospholipase A_2 activity is associated with risk of coronary heart disease and ischemic stroke: the Rotterdam Study. *Circulation*, **111**, 570–75.

[62] Koenig, W., Khuseyinova, N., Lowel, H. *et al.* (2004) Lipoprotein-associated phospholipase A_2 adds to risk prediction of incident coronary events by C-reactive protein in apparently healthy middle-aged men from the general population: results from the 14-year follow-up of a large cohort from southern Germany. *Circulation*, **110**, 1903–8.

[63] Blake, G.J., Dada, N., Fox, J.C. *et al.* (2001) A prospective evaluation of lipoprotein-associated phospholipase A(2) levels and the risk of future cardiovascular events in women. *Journal of the American College of Cardiology*, **38**, 1302–6.

[64] Corsetti, J.P., Rainwater, D.L., Moss, A.J. *et al.* (2006) High lipoprotein-associated phospholipase A_2 is a risk factor for recurrent coronary events in postinfarction patients. *Clinical Chemistry*, **52**, 1331–38.

[65] Tselepis, A.D. and John Chapman, M. (2002) Inflammation, bioactive lipids and atherosclerosis: potential roles of a lipoprotein-associated phospholipase A_2, platelet activating factor-acetylhydrolase. *Atherosclerosis Supplements*, **3**, 57–68.

[66] Caslake, M.J. and Packard, C.J. (2003) Lipoprotein-associated phospholipase A_2 (platelet-activating factor acetylhydrolase) and cardiovascular disease. *Current Opinion in Lipidology*, **14**, 347–52.

[67] Karabina, S.A., Liapikos, T.A., Grekas, G. *et al.* (1994) Distribution of PAF-acetylhydrolase activity in human plasma low-density lipoprotein subfractions. *Biochimica et Biophysica Acta*, **1**, 34–38.

[68] Murugesan, G., Sandhya Rani, M.R., Gerber, C.E. *et al.* (2003) Lysophosphatidylcholine regulates human microvascular endothelial cell expression of chemokines. *Journal of Molecular and Cellular Cardiology*, **35**, 1375–84.

[69] Chaudhuri, P., Colles, S.M., Damron, D.S. and Graham, L.M. (2003) Lysophosphatidylcholine inhibits endothelial cell migration by increasing intracellular calcium and activating calpain. *Arteriosclerosis, Thrombosis and Vascular Biology*, **23**, 218–23.

[70] Zalewski, A. and Macphee, C. (2005) Role of lipoprotein-associated phospholipase A$_2$ in atherosclerosis: biology, epidemiology, and possible therapeutic target. *Arteriosclerosis, Thrombosis and Vascular Biology*, **25**, 923–31.

[71] Lanman, R.B., Wolfert, R.L., Fleming, J.K. *et al.* (2006) Lipoprotein-associated phospholipase A$_2$: review and recommendation of a clinical cut point for adults. *Preventive Cardiology*, **9**, 138–43.

[72] Kolodgie, F.D., Burke, A.P., Skorija, K.S. *et al.* (2006) Lipoprotein-associated phospholipase A$_2$ protein expression in the natural progression of human coronary atherosclerosis. *Arteriosclerosis, Thrombosis and Vascular Biology*, **26**, 2523–29.

[73] Marcovina, S.M., Koschinsky, M.L., Albers, J.J. and Skarlatos, S. (2003) Report of the National Heart, Lung, and Blood Institute Workshop on Lipoprotein(a) and Cardiovascular Disease: recent advances and future directions. *Clinical Chemistry*, **49**, 1785–96.

[74] Marcovina, S.M. and Koschinsky, M.L. (2003) Evaluation of lipoprotein(a) as a prothrombotic factor: progress from bench to bedside. *Current Opinion in Lipidology*, **14**, 361–66.

[75] Berg, K. (1963) A new serum type system in man – the LP system. *Acta Pathologica et Microbiologica Scandinavica*, **59**, 369–82.

[76] Jones, G.T., van Rij, A.M., Cole, J. *et al.* (2007) Plasma lipoprotein(a) indicates risk for 4 distinct forms of vascular disease. *Clinical Chemistry*, **53**, 679–85.

[77] Rath, M., Niendorf, A., Reblin, T. *et al.* (1989) Detection and quantification of lipoprotein(a) in the arterial wall of 107 coronary bypass patients. [erratum appears in Arteriosclerosis 1990 Nov–Dec;10(6):1147]. *Arteriosclerosis*, **9**, 579–92.

[78] Dangas, G., Mehran, R., Harpel, P.C. *et al.* (1998) Lipoprotein(a) and inflammation in human coronary atheroma: association with the severity of clinical presentation. *Journal of the American College of Cardiology*, **32**, 2035–42.

[79] Danesh, J., Whincup, P., Walker, M. *et al.* (2000) Low grade inflammation and coronary heart disease: prospective study and updated meta-analyses. *British Medical Journal*, **321**, 199–204.

[80] Sandholzer, C., Hallman, D.M., Saha, N. *et al.* (1991) Effects of the apolipoprotein(a) size polymorphism on the lipoprotein(a) concentration in 7 ethnic groups. *Human Genetics*, **86**, 607–14.

[81] Boerwinkle, E., Leffert, C.C., Lin, J. *et al.* (1992) Apolipoprotein(a) gene accounts for greater than 90% of the variation in plasma lipoprotein(a) concentrations. *Journal of Clinical Investigation*, **90**, 52–60.

[82] McKenney, J.M., Jones, P.H., Bays, H.E. *et al.* (2007) Comparative effects on lipid levels of combination therapy with a statin and extended-release niacin or ezetimibe versus a statin alone (the COMPELL study). *Atherosclerosis*, **192**, 432–37.

[83] Pan, J., Van, J.T., Chan, E. *et al.* (2002) Extended-release niacin treatment of the atherogenic lipid profile and lipoprotein(a) in diabetes. *Metabolism: Clinical and Experimental*, **51**, 1120–127.

[84] Pan, J., Lin, M., Kesala, R.L. *et al.* (2002) Niacin treatment of the atherogenic lipid profile and Lp(a) in diabetes. *Diabetes, Obesity and Metabolism*, **4**, 255–61.

[85] Marcovina, S.M., Koschinsky, M.L., Albers, J.J. and Skarlatos, S. (2003) Report of the National Heart, Lung, and Blood Institute Workshop on Lipoprotein(a) and Cardiovascular Disease: recent advances and future directions. *Clinical Chemistry*, **49**, 1785–96.

[86] Maron, B.A.L.J. (2007) Should hyperhomocysteinemia be treated in patients with atherosclerotic disease? *Current Atherosclerosis Reports*, **9**, 375–83.

[87] Tran, H., Hankey, G.J. and Eikelboom, J.W. (2006) Homocysteine – should we screen and treat in preventive cardiology programs? *Journal of Cardiopulmonary Rehabilitation*, **26**, 281–87.

[88] Liao, D., Tan, H., Hui, R. *et al.* (2006) Hyperhomocysteinemia decreases circulating high-density lipoprotein by inhibiting apolipoprotein A-I protein synthesis and enhancing HDL cholesterol clearance. *Circulation Research*, **99**, 598–606.

[89] Selhub, J., Jacques, P.F., Wilson, P.W. *et al.* (1993) Vitamin status and intake as primary determinants of homocysteinemia in an elderly population. *Journal of the American Medical Association*, **270**, 2693–98.

[90] Welch, G.N. and Loscalzo, J. (1998) Homocysteine and atherothrombosis. *The New England Journal of Medicine*, **338**, 1042–50.

[91] Kang, S.S., Wong, P.W. and Malinow, M.R. (1992) Hyperhomocyst(e)inemia as a risk factor for occlusive vascular disease. *Annual Review of Nutrition*, **12**, 279–98.

[92] Wierzbicki, A.S. (2007) Homocysteine and cardiovascular disease: a review of the evidence. *Diabetes and Vascular Disease Research*, **4**, 143–50.

[93] Ridker, P.M., Manson, J.E., Buring, J.E. *et al.* (1999) Homocysteine and risk of cardiovascular disease among postmenopausal women. *Journal of the American Medical Association*, **281**, 1817–21.

[94] Bonaa, K.H., Njolstad, I., Ueland, P.M. *et al.* (2006) Homocysteine lowering and cardiovascular events after acute myocardial infarction. *The New England Journal of Medicine*, **354**, 1578–88.

[95] Carlsson, C.M. (2006) Homocysteine lowering with folic acid and vitamin B supplements: effects on cardiovascular disease in older adults. *Drugs and Aging*, **23**, 491–502.

[96] Lonn, E., Yusuf, S., Arnold, M.J. *et al.* (2006) Homocysteine lowering with folic acid and B vitamins in vascular disease. *The New England Journal of Medicine*, **354**, 1567–77.

[97] Toole, J.F., Malinow, M.R., Chambless, L.E. *et al.* (2004) Lowering homocysteine in patients with ischemic stroke to prevent recurrent stroke, myocardial infarction, and death: the Vitamin Intervention for Stroke Prevention (VISP) randomized controlled trial. *Journal of the American Medical Association*, **291**, 565–75.

[98] Lange, H., Suryapranata, H., De Luca, G. *et al.* (2004) Folate therapy and in-stent restenosis after coronary stenting. *The New England Journal of Medicine*, **350**, 2673–81.

[99] MacMahon, M., Kirkpatrick, C., Cummings, C.E. *et al.* (2000) A pilot study with simvastatin and folic acid/vitamin B12 in preparation for the Study of the Effectiveness of Additional Reductions in Cholesterol and Homocysteine (SEARCH). *Nutrition Metabolism and Cardiovascular Diseases*, **10**, 195–203.

[100] Cromwell, W.C. and Otvos, J.D. (2004) Low-density lipoprotein particle number and risk for cardiovascular disease. *Current Atherosclerosis Reports*, **6**, 381–87.
[101] Kuller, L., Arnold, A., Tracy, R. *et al.* (2002) Nuclear magnetic resonance spectroscopy of lipoproteins and risk of coronary heart disease in the cardiovascular health study. *Arteriosclerosis, Thrombosis and Vascular Biology*, **22**, 1175–80.
[102] Blake, G.J., Otvos, J.D., Rifai, N. and Ridker, P.M. (2002) Low-density lipoprotein particle concentration and size as determined by nuclear magnetic resonance spectroscopy as predictors of cardiovascular disease in women. *Circulation*, **106**, 1930–37.
[103] Mackey, R.H., Kuller, L.H., Sutton-Tyrrell, K. *et al.* (2002) Lipoprotein subclasses and coronary artery calcium in postmenopausal women from the healthy women study. *American Journal of Cardiology*, **90**, 17.

10 A Primer on Clinical Trials and Critical Review of Clinical Trial Reports for the Clinician

Key Points

- *The randomized, controlled trial remains the 'gold standard' for evaluation of medical interventions.*

- *A number of issues should be addressed in order for a trial to produce valid and generalizable results including: appropriate selection of study participants, random subject assignment to treatments, blinding and use of a placebo where practical.*

- *Potential problems can occur during study conduct such as poor subject compliance, excessive or differential dropout, incomplete blinding, and changes in treatment during the trial that may confound the interpretation of the influence of the intervention.*

- *In order to interpret clinical trial results, three factors should be assessed: chance (random variation), bias (a nonrandom error that results in an incorrect estimate of a treatment effect), and confounding (the possibility that an observed association between a treatment and the response is due to the effects of differences between the treatment groups other than the treatment under study).*

The randomized clinical trial is universally accepted as the most reliable method for evaluating the efficacy and safety of medical treatments. Although commonly applied to drug therapies, the clinical trial process can also be used to evaluate medical devices, surgical procedures, lifestyle

Practical Lipid Management: Concepts and Controversies   Peter P. Toth and Kevin C. Maki
© 2008 John Wiley & Sons, Ltd

interventions, and policy options. One famous example of the latter was the Newburgh–Kingston dental caries study. In that trial, one entire community was randomly allocated to have fluoride added to the drinking water supply while the other did not [1]. The results showed large reductions in the development of dental caries in the community with the fluoridated water (Newburgh) compared with the community that did not receive supplemented water (Kingston).

The central tenets for the conduct of clinical trials were not widely understood or practiced before the 1950s, when Sir Austin Bradford Hill published a series of articles on the proper conduct of clinical experiments [2]. These papers emphasized the value of such fundamental concepts as the use of random allocation to treatments, concurrent controls, clearly defined inclusion and exclusion criteria, a defined treatment protocol, and statistical methods for separating treatment effects from random variation. Surprisingly, prior to the 1960s, no formal requirements for clinical trial evaluation were in place before a drug could be marketed in the USA. The discovery that thalidomide produced birth defects in the children of pregnant women who had taken the drug as an antiemetic and/or sleep aid led to formal requirements for clinical trial evaluation of new drug products, and it was not until 1969 that submission of data from randomized, controlled trials was mandatory for receiving marketing approval for a new drug from the United States Food and Drug Administration.

10.1   DESIGN ISSUES AFFECTING THE VALIDITY AND GENERALIZABILITY OF CLINICAL TRIAL RESULTS

Although properly conducted randomized, controlled clinical trials represent the "gold standard" for evaluation of medical interventions, a number of issues must be satisfactorily addressed in order for a trial to produce valid and generalizable results. Of particular interest to the clinician are the study entry criteria, characteristics of the study population, compliance with the treatment regimen and potential sources of bias or confounding that might influence interpretation and application of the results in medical practice.

SELECTION OF STUDY PARTICIPANTS

The selection of study participants has important implications for the interpretation of the study results and their generalizability to the clinical setting. Often a trial will have strict entry criteria, which may be ideal for minimizing variability in response, thus enhancing the power of the trial to detect differences between treatments, but may also lead to a study sample that is not representative of patients typically encountered in clinical practice. It is not uncommon for a trial to exclude 70% or more of subjects screened. For example, the Dietary Approaches to Stop Hypertension (DASH) trial screened 8813 subjects in order to identify 459 who were ultimately randomized to the three treatment arms (5.2% of those screened) [3]. While the results from the DASH trial have subsequently been replicated, lending support to the validity of the study results (which showed that a diet low in fat with above-average intakes of fruits, vegetables, and low-fat dairy products could lower blood pressure), caution is warranted regarding the impact that might be expected in clinical practice with such an intervention, given that only one in 20 subjects screened ultimately qualified and was willing to enter the treatment phase.

It is important for the clinician not to view clinical trial results in isolation. Systematic review papers are useful to help the clinician assess consistency of results across trials and to confirm the robustness of findings from trials in samples drawn from different populations [4]. Early statin trials showed the usefulness of these drugs for reducing coronary heart disease morbidity, but left important questions unanswered regarding efficacy in subgroups such as women, the elderly, those with diabetes and other conditions such as hypertension and heart failure. It has taken years to develop a body of trial literature to sufficiently address statin efficacy in many of these subgroups.

Volunteerism and study entry criteria may influence participation in ways that produce important differences between those who are willing and eligible to participate in a trial and those who are not. Morbidity and mortality in the placebo groups of clinical endpoint trials has been consistently reported to be lower than that in the general population. This may result in part from the greater frequency of contact with medical professionals during the trial, allowing early warning signs to be detected more readily. However, it may also result from differences between participants and nonparticipants due to study exclusion criteria (those at the greatest risk may be excluded) and the fact that people willing to expend the time and effort required to participate in trials tend to be more health conscious and more compliant with treatment regimens than average. Another factor that may influence outcomes in the opposite direction is that one motivating factor for participation in a trial is the medical care that is provided as part of the trial at no charge. This may be more of an inducement to participate for people lacking health insurance or in lower socioeconomic strata than more affluent individuals. Lower socioeconomic status is well known to be associated with a number of adverse health outcomes [5–7].

Baseline characteristics of subjects may markedly influence response, which could have important implications for generalizability of clinical trial

results. For example, today, the predominant view among clinicians is that
statins produce modest favorable changes in triglyceride and high-density
lipoprotein cholesterol (HDL-C) concentrations, whereas fibrates produce
much larger effects on these variables. However, careful evaluation of
the results from published trials reveals that statins produce much greater
reductions in triglycerides and increases in HDL-C among subjects who
are hypertriglyceridemic than is the case for normotriglyceridemic subjects. Comparing results from studies of statin and fibrate treatments in
hyptertriglyceridemic subjects suggests that moderate doses of statins produce changes in triglycerides and HDL-C that are only slightly less than
those observed with fibrate therapy in those with hypertriglyceridemia. An
example of such a comparison is shown in Figure 10.1, which shows results
from trials in which one of the authors (KCM) was directly involved. Since
statins lower low-density lipoprotein cholesterol (LDL-C) to a larger degree,
moderate doses of drugs such as atorvastatin, rosuvastatin, and simvastatin
appear to produce larger reductions in non-HDL-C than is the case for
the marketed doses of fibrate drugs. Unfortunately, published results from

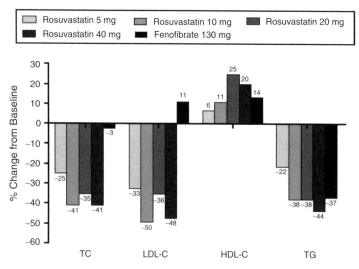

Figure 10.1   Placebo-corrected changes in total cholesterol (TC), low-density
lipoprotein cholesterol (LDL-C), high-density lipoprotein cholesterol (HDL-C), and
triglycerides (TG) in subjects with hypertriglyceridemia (baseline TG 300-799 in
the rosuvastatin study and 300-999 in the fenofibrate study). Adapted from package
inserts for Crestor (rosuvastatin) and Antara (fenofibrate).

large studies directly comparing the effects of statins and fibrates on the serum lipid profile and cardiovascular outcomes are lacking. Nevertheless, this example illustrates the difficulties that can arise in comparing responses to drugs across groups with differing baseline characteristics (in this case baseline lipid concentrations) and the resulting difficulties in generalization of trial results to clinical practice.

THE IMPORTANCE OF RANDOM TREATMENT ALLOCATION

The medical literature is replete with examples of treatments that generated great enthusiasm based on observational data or nonrandomized clinical studies which were later found to be of little or no value when evaluated in carefully designed and executed randomized clinical trials. Random assignment to treatments so that the investigator cannot anticipate which treatment the next subject will receive minimizes known and unrecognized sources of bias and confounding that could impact the study results.

Assignment to treatment using a method in which the investigator can anticipate the next treatment such as alternating active and control, or assigning to active on odd days and control on even days, is likely to lead to unintentional, or even intentional, bias in treatment allocation. If a clinician believes in the efficacy of a treatment, she may be more apt to assign a potential subject to an active arm who has a more severe form of the disease or, conversely, if someone has a more severe case of the condition under study and the clinician believes the subject is unlikely to benefit from the treatment, she may be more likely to "save that slot" for someone who is believed to be more likely to benefit.

With a large enough sample, equal distribution across treatment groups of characteristics related to treatment response is highly likely. In smaller studies, a stratified randomization scheme is sometimes used for variables that are expected to be associated with treatment response. With this approach, subjects are first segregated into cells based on the characteristic (e.g. cells for those with and without diabetes) and then random assignment takes place within each cell. This does not guarantee equal numbers of subjects with and without the characteristic in the overall study sample, but eliminates the possibility of a substantial imbalance between treatments for subjects with that characteristic. For instance, subjects with diabetes may make up only 10% of the study sample. Thus, if a trial has two arms, active and control, and a subset of 80 subjects with diabetes is randomized, roughly 40 will be assigned to each treatment, with no possibility of allocating 60 subjects with diabetes to one group or the other.

BLINDING AND USE OF A PLACEBO ARE DESIRABLE, BUT NOT ALWAYS POSSIBLE

Blinding refers to masking of the study subjects, investigators and other study staff to the treatment that a subject is actually receiving. A single-blind study is typically one in which the subjects are blinded to treatment allocation, but the study staff are not, and a double-blind study is one in which both the subjects and the investigators (and other evaluators) are blinded to the treatment assignment. This insures that neither the study subjects nor those evaluating efficacy and tolerability are biased in their assessments. Blinding is particularly important when the assessment of response has a subjective component, such when assessing therapies for conditions such as arthritis pain, migraine headaches, anxiety disorders, menopausal symptoms, premenstrual syndromes, etc. The psychological effect of receiving a therapy, even if there is a chance it is a placebo, should not be underestimated. Regression to the mean undoubtedly plays some role, that is, people are more likely to enroll when their symptoms are at their worst and tend to improve whether or not they receive the active treatment. Nevertheless, it has been striking to the authors that the responses in the placebo groups of studies evaluating treatments for conditions such as arthritis [8] and menopausal vasomotor symptoms [9] regularly show improvements of 30–60%. Thus, readers should be very suspicious of studies with subjective outcomes where adequate blinding is not employed.

At times, ethical considerations influence whether blinding or use of a placebo control is desirable. Once the efficacy of a treatment becomes sufficiently well demonstrated, it becomes unethical to withhold the treatment from those who could benefit for any substantial length of time. For this reason, placebo-controlled studies of drugs for hypercholesterolemia, diabetes, and hypertension that last for more than a few weeks, particularly in high risk subjects, are a thing of the past. This results in the requirement to demonstrate that new therapies are "noninferior" to existing therapies or that they produce added benefits. Such questions generally require much larger sample sizes than is the case for placebo-controlled studies.

For some surgical procedure studies, subjects are randomly assigned to receive one procedure or another, or even to receive the actual procedure or a sham procedure in which an incision is made, but the surgical procedure under study is not completed. In some cases, the risk and expense associated with a sham procedure are considered too great to make this option viable. For example, the Clinical Outcomes Utilizing Revascularization and Aggressive Drug Evaluation (COURAGE) trial compared optimal medical therapy with and without percutaneous coronary intervention in subjects with stable coronary artery disease and evidence of myocardial ischemia [10]. Since subjects in the group receiving optimal medical therapy alone did not undergo a sham procedure, they were aware of their treatment assignment. However, all events were adjudicated by a committee of experts that were blinded to treatment assignment in order to minimize potential bias introduced by lack of blinding.

POTENTIAL PROBLEMS WITH STUDY CONDUCT THAT MAY INFLUENCE VALIDITY OR GENERALIZABILITY

Several issues may arise during the conduct of a trial that have the potential to impact the validity and/or generalizability of the trial results. These include such issues as poor subject compliance, excessive or differential dropout, incomplete blinding, and changes in treatment during the trial that confound the study results.

In order for a trial to produce valid results, it is necessary for subjects to adhere to the treatment regimen. Some trials are so complex, and create such a subject burden, that a large proportion of subjects do not comply well with the study protocol. When this occurs, it will tend to bias the results toward a finding of no effect for the treatment under study. An example was the landmark Lipid Research Clinics Coronary Primary Prevention Trial (LRC-CPPT) in which subjects were randomly assigned to receive cholestyramine (a bile acid sequestrant) or placebo. Because of the unpleasant texture and gastrointestinal side effects produced by the study drug, many subjects were not fully compliant. A subgroup analysis showed that while the drug was effective overall, those who were most compliant had the largest reductions in cholesterol levels and the greatest reduction in event risk, suggesting that the full potential benefit of treatment may have been underestimated [11].

A related problem is excessive dropout, which may occur when the treatment has unpleasant side effects or when the treatment regimen and/or study procedures are excessively burdensome. Two types of investigations that are known for their problems with high dropout rates are weight loss and smoking cessation trials. A further complicating factor is that dropout may be differential. Subjects in whom the treatment is effective may be more likely to stay in the study, while those for whom the treatment is not working well may be more apt to drop out. Problems arise if differential dropout occurs between active and control conditions. Various statistical techniques are available that attempt to minimize the potential bias associated with differential dropout, but none are fully satisfactory. Differential dropout can affect the results in a way that favors the treatment (e.g. higher dropout among those for whom the treatment is ineffective) or the control condition (e.g. higher dropout in the active group when side effects are more common or more severe among those in whom the treatment is most effective). It may also be difficult or impossible to determine the outcome (e.g. cardiovascular events) for subjects who drop out of a trial, which may cause the investigation to have insufficient statistical power to detect differences between treatments that would have been detectable with accumulation of a sufficient number of events during the treatment period to show statistically significant differences between treatments. Clinicians should be aware of the potential for dropout to influence results and carefully read the Discussion section of any clinical trial publication for the authors' views on the possible influence of dropout on the interpretation of the results.

Sometimes complete blinding is difficult or impossible. For example, if a drug has characteristic side effects, many subjects assigned to active treatment will know that they are not on the placebo. Examples include flushing from niacin and altered menstrual bleeding patterns associated with sex hormone therapies. In such cases, innovative solutions have sometimes been employed to minimize the possibility of bias. In some trials, a very small and nonefficacious quantity of niacin was included in the placebo product so that subjects assigned to placebo would experience mild flushing. In the Heart and Estrogen/Progestin Replacement Study (HERS), separate evaluators were employed to assess gynecological and nongynecological issues in order to minimize bias that might occur due to knowledge of vaginal bleeding that would only be expected to occur among the women assigned to the active treatment [12].

One of the authors has been involved in the design and conduct of hundreds of clinical trials. His favorite story illustrating how difficult it is at times to maintain complete blinding involved a study of a product that changed the color of subjects' urine. Although great effort was expended to insure that the active and placebo tablets were identical with regard to sensory characteristics, the author was dismayed to hear subjects in the lobby of his clinic discussing urine color and guessing which study product each was taking based on these changes (or lack thereof).

During clinical outcomes trials that have extended follow-up periods, changes in treatment may confound the study results. The classic example of this phenomenon was the Multiple Risk Factor Intervention Trial (MR-FIT) in which subjects were assigned to receive aggressive multiple risk factor modification or standard care. Over the extended follow-up period (six to eight years), standard care changed in such a way that narrowed the differences between the treatment arms in levels of several cardiovascular disease risk factors. As a result, the observed differences between the groups were less than targeted and the trial failed to show a significant difference in the primary outcome variable of mortality from coronary heart disease and all causes [13]. Later studies confirmed the efficacy of risk factor management for reducing cardiovascular morbidity and mortality.

A more recent example of changing medical practice influencing the results of a trial was the Fenofibrate Intervention and Event Lowering in Diabetes (FIELD) trial. Subjects with type 2 diabetes ($n = 9795$) were randomly assigned to receive fenofibrate 200 mg day^{-1} or placebo and followed for an average of approximately five years [14]. The investigators had assumed that some subjects in both groups would receive ad_____ lipid-altering therapy during the study because their personal physicians would be dissatisfied with participants' lipid control. They assumed that there would be slightly more such subjects in the placebo group. However, during the follow-up period, more than twice as many subjects received additional lipid-altering therapy (statins) in the placebo group compared with the fenofibrate group (17 vs 8%). This was particularly true among subjects with preexisting coronary heart disease. As a result, the differences in blood lipid parameters narrowed over the treatment period. The study failed to show a significant difference in its primary endpoint, coronary heart disease death or nonfatal myocardial infarction (a nonsignificant 11% reduction was observed in the fenofibrate group, $p = 0.16$). Interpretation of the study results is confounded by the differential use of statin therapy, rendering the clinical implications of the results of this large and expensive investigation uncertain. It is tempting to speculate that if the differences in lipid levels that prevailed during the first four months of the trial had persisted throughout, the difference between groups in the primary outcome variable may have been larger and statistically significant. Investigators designing future studies will need to include strategies to minimize or avoid this problem.

10.2 CHANCE, BIAS, AND CONFOUNDING AS POTENTIAL EXPLANATIONS FOR TRIAL RESULTS

The interpretation of clinical trial results involves assessing the degree to which three factors: (i) chance, (ii) bias, and (iii) confounding, may explain the observed difference (or lack of difference) in responses and/or outcomes between treatments.

CHANCE (RANDOM VARIATION) AS A POSSIBLE EXPLANATION FOR AN OBSERVED RESULT

If two groups differ numerically in their response to a treatment, one of the first questions asked is usually: "What was the p value?" A p value represents an assessment of the probability that an observed difference could have occurred due to random variation. Traditionally, a p value less than 0.05 is considered "statistical significant". If the p value for a statistical comparison between two treatments is 0.04, for instance, this indicates that there is a 4% chance that a difference of the magnitude observed could have occurred by chance. The smaller the p value, the lower the likelihood that a given difference occurred due to random variation. A p value of 0.001 indicates that there is only a 1 in 1000 (0.1%) probability that the observed difference is due to random variation.

Confidence intervals are related to p values. They provide a measure of the precision of an estimate for a difference between treatments in a clinical trial. Typically those included in published papers are 95% confidence intervals, although 90 or 99% confidence intervals are sometimes presented. The 95% confidence interval is the range of values in which one can be 95% certain that the true value for a point estimate lies (e.g. a mean, a rate, or a risk ratio). Thus, if a difference between groups in LDL-C response is −35% with a confidence interval from −55 to −15%, this indicates that one can be 95% certain that the true mean difference lies between the range of −55 to −15%. Another way to state this is that if the trial were repeated 100 times, it would be expected that 95% of the mean differences would fall in the range of −55 to −15%.

If a 95% confidence interval crosses zero for the difference between treatments, this indicates that the difference was not statistically significant at the 5% level, that is, the p value is >0.05, and one cannot rule out a difference of zero with 95% confidence. Where treatments are being compared using ratio statistics such as a relative risk, odds ratio, or hazard ratio, the p value will be significant if the 95% confidence interval does not include 1.0. For example, as discussed above, in the FIELD trial, the hazard ratio for coronary heart disease events was 0.89 with a 95% confidence interval that ranged from 0.75 to 1.05, $p = 0.16$. This indicates that the hazard for an event in the fenofibrate group was 89% of that in the placebo group (lower by 11%). However, because the 95% confidence interval crosses 1.0, it is clear that this difference was not statistically significant at the 5% level, as confirmed by a p value of 0.16.

Figure 10.2 shows a summary of the results from the Collaborative AtoRvastatin Diabetes Study (CARDS) [15]. The trial showed a significant difference between the atorvastatin and placebo groups for the primary endpoint of time to first occurrence of a composite variable that included acute coronary heart disease events, coronary revascularization, or stroke. The hazard ratio for the primary endpoint showed a significant ($p = 0.001$) reduction of 37% (hazard ratio = 0.63), with a 95% confidence interval of 0.48–0.83 that did not include zero. However, for death from any cause, the hazard ratio was 0.73 with a 95% confidence interval of 0.52–1.01. Because the confidence interval crosses zero, this indicates that the observed 27% reduction in mortality was not significant at the 5% level, as confirmed by a p value of 0.059.

One issue that clinicians should keep in mind is that when many hypotheses are tested, it should be expected that a few will show "statistical significance" by chance. One of the authors once worked with a colleague to write a program to run a simulated coin flipping experiment. The probability of flipping heads or tails was exactly 50%. A series of 100 sets of 100 coin

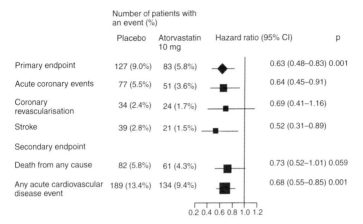

Figure 10.2 Effects of treatment on primary and secondary endpoints in the Collaborative AtoRvastatin Diabetes Study (CARDS). CARDS was a trial evaluating treatment with atorvastatin vs. placebo for primary prevention of cardiovascular events in 2338 subjects with type 2 diabetes. From Colhoun, H.M. *et al.* (2004) *Lancet*, **364**, 685–96, [15].

flips were simulated. In 5 of the 100 sets, the observed value for heads differed "significantly" from 50% with a p value <0.05. Actual values for percent heads ranged from 38 to 61%. This experiment illustrates very nicely that if one runs 100 statistical tests, it should not be unexpected that about 5% will show p values <0.05 by chance.

For this reason, it is important that a single primary outcome variable (or small number of variables) is clearly prespecified in advance. Significant comparisons from secondary and subgroup analyses should be interpreted with caution, particularly if the p value for a comparison is close to 0.05. It is not uncommon for as many as 100 or more statistical comparisons to be made in a single trial dataset. Such nonprimary comparisons can be very useful for generating hypotheses, but should be viewed cautiously until replicated in additional trials specifically designed to test those hypotheses. Even significant results for primary outcome variables should not be taken as definitive until a body of literature grows demonstrating consistency of results across trials. One should always remember that no matter how large the difference, and how small the p value, very low-probability differences do occasionally occur due to chance. Therefore, results from clinical trials should always be interpreted in the context of the totality of evidence from all available sources, including other clinical trials, results from observational studies, and other information such as animal and mechanistic studies.

When reading a report of clinical trial results, one should also keep in mind the concept of statistical power. Failure to detect a significant difference between treatments could be a consequence of there being no clinically important effect. Alternatively, a nonsignificant p value may have occurred because the study lacked sufficient statistical power to detect an effect that is clinically meaningful. A thorough discussion of statistical power is beyond the scope of this chapter. However, the central idea is that power is increased with a greater number of subjects, greater precision in the measurement for continuous variables (e.g. lipid levels), a larger treatment effect, and a greater number of events for trials comparing risks for onset of a disease or condition (e.g. cardiovascular events). For this reason, trials sometimes need to be extended beyond their originally planned follow-up period because an insufficient number of events have accumulated to reliably evaluate the intervention. Conversely, some trials are stopped early because enough events have accumulated to demonstrate benefit, lack of benefit, or even harm, earlier than anticipated.

BIAS AND CONFOUNDING

Bias and confounding have already been discussed in the context of issues that can arise during a trial (e.g. incomplete blinding, poor compliance, excessive, or differential dropout) that make interpretation of the study results more difficult. Bias is defined as a systematic error that results in an incorrect estimate of a treatment effect, such as differential compliance or dropout. Confounding involves the possibility that an observed association between a treatment and the response is due to the effects of differences between the treatment groups other than the treatment under study. The FIELD trial was provided as an example where differences between the treatment groups in the addition of statin therapy to the study treatment (fenofibrate or placebo) were present, confounding the interpretation of the results. Another confounding factor that sometimes arises is baseline differences between groups, despite random allocation to treatments. If the primary outcome variable is coronary heart disease events and the treatment groups differ with regard to Framingham risk score at baseline, this would be a potential confounding factor and the investigators would need to carefully examine the results to evaluate the degree to which such confounding may have influenced the final results.

10.3   EFFICACY VERSUS EFFECTIVENESS

Efficacy refers to whether an intervention produces the desired effects when properly implemented under controlled conditions; whereas effectiveness refers to whether an intervention is typically successful in clinical practice [16]. In order for a treatment to be useful, it must be both efficacious and effective.

The primary statistical analysis for most clinical trials is conducted on an "intention-to-treat" basis. This means that all subjects randomly assigned to receive a treatment are included in the analysis. Subjects are then treated in the analysis as being part of their assigned group, whether or not they actually received the treatment, adhered to the treatment regimen, or even received the opposite treatment. Thus, the analysis follows the intended treatment (i.e., the intention to treat), regardless of whether or how well the intervention was actually carried out. Frequently, a secondary "per protocol" analysis is completed in which subjects who discontinued or who had material protocol violations, including poor adherence, are excluded from the analysis.

When the results from intention-to-treat and per protocol analyses agree, this provides some reassurance that the results obtained in clinical practice are likely to be similar to those reported in the trial (at least for similar groups of patients). However, the clinician should be wary of results from trials in which only a per protocol analysis is presented, as these may be biased [17]. For instance, if subjects with poor prognosis are less likely to be able to adhere to the treatment regimen, a per protocol analysis will exclude the least compliant subjects, who are also those with the worst prognosis. This may result in an overestimation of the effect of the intervention. In addition, treatments with unpleasant side effects, such as some early lipid drugs (e.g. first generation bile acid sequestrants and immediate release niacin) were often associated with poor compliance. Eliminating subjects with poor compliance from the analysis would provide a distorted picture of the clinical utility of the medications. Conversely, the "intention-to-treat" analysis may underestimate the degree to which a highly compliant patient might benefit. Therefore, it is instructive to examine the degree to which intention-to-treat and per protocol analyses results differ, when both are presented, as this may provide clues regarding how well the intervention might be expected to perform in clinical practice.

10.4 USEFUL QUESTIONS TO ASK WHEN EVALUATING A PUBLISHED CLINICAL TRIAL REPORT

The following are questions the clinician may use to systematically evaluate many of the most common issues that affect the interpretation of clinical trial results. These questions cover each of the main points covered in this chapter.

1. Was the subject sample similar to patients commonly observed in clinical practice? If not, might strict entry criteria limit generalizability of the results?

2. Were important subgroups represented (e.g. both sexes, smokers, those with obesity and/or diabetes, various lipid phenotypes)? If so, were responses similar in these subgroups?

3. Were random allocation, concurrent controls and blinding all present? If not, why and how might these issues affect the results?

4. Were subjects generally compliant with the treatment regimen? Was compliance consistent between treatments?

5. Did the trial suffer from excessive subject attrition or differential dropout between treatments?

6. Was the primary outcome variable prespecified and clearly stated?

7. Did the trial show a statistically significant difference for the primary outcome variable?

8. Did the results appear consistent across subgroups and secondary analyses?

9. If significant results were not achieved, could this have been due to the trial lacking sufficient statistical power to detect a clinically meaningful difference (e.g. secondary to a sample size that was too small, high variability in the response, excessive dropout or an unexpectedly low event rate)?

10. How do the results from this trial align with those from other sources (clinical trials, observational studies, animal experiments, and mechanistic investigations)?

CONTROVERSY

SHOULD LIPID DRUGS BE APPROVED WITHOUT CLINICAL EVENT DATA?

In recent years, issues have arisen regarding adverse effects of several classes of medication on cardiovascular event risk. Rofecoxib (Vioxx) was withdrawn from the market due to an unanticipated increase cardiovascular events, and warnings were added to other similar drugs regarding effects on cardiovascular events [1, 2]. The development of muraglitazar (a peroxisome proliferator activated receptor-alpha/gamma agonist) and torcetrapib (a cholesteryl ester transfer protein inhibitor) were discontinued due to greater cardiovascular event risk compared with placebo or other compounds for the same indication

[3, 4]. In addition, the FDA reviewed concerns regarding rosiglita-zone (Avandia®, a peroxisome proliferator activated receptor-gamma agonist) and possible increased risk of cardiovascular events in 2007. On 30 July 2007, the FDA's Endocrine and Metabolic Advisory Committee and the Drug Safety and Risk Management Advisory Committee recommended that rosiglitazone continue to be marketed, and further recommended that information be added to the labeling for risk of heart attacks (ischemic risks) [5].

These incidents have prompted some to advocate additional safety testing beyond what has traditionally been required for drug approval. A great deal of debate is ongoing about what the standards should be for approval of drugs intended to alter lipid metabolism and/or retard atherosclerosis. Some argue that drugs for these indications should not be approved until their effects on event risk have been demonstrated. However, such studies take years and many millions of dollars to conduct. The consequences of such a requirement might be to inhibit the development of innovative new therapies in these areas because of the high cost, and to potentially delay the avail-ability of new, effective therapies for a period of years, resulting in unnecessary morbidity and mortality that might have been avoided had the drug been available. The incremental human and financial costs associated with more stringent testing requirements are difficult to quantify, making cost to benefit comparisons of different policy approaches difficult to analyze.

The FDA has historically taken a position on this issue that the authors feel is reasonable, but imperfect. For drugs that primarily act to lower LDL-C and other atherogenic lipoproteins, only the standard drug safety trials and evidence of favorable effects on accepted bio-chemical surrogate markers have been required. Accepted biochem-ical markers include LDL-C, non-HDL-C and Apo B. In agreement with the National Cholesterol Education Panel Adult Treatment Panel III (NCEP ATP III) guidelines, changes in triglyceride and HDL-C concentrations are considered, but as secondary outcomes, providing supportive evidence of efficacy. Examples of drugs that have received approval based on these surrogate measures in the past several years include colesevelam (Welchol®, a bile acid sequestrant) and ezetim-ibe (Zetia®, a cholesterol absorption inhibitor). Given the strong and consistent evidence of benefit from lowering atherogenic lipoproteins through various types of interventions, including several classes of medication, diet and ileal bypass, the authors agree that a reasonable assumption of benefit can be inferred from such trials.

For other classes of medications, such as those intended to primarily influence HDL-C or the progression of atherosclerosis through various mechanisms, the FDA position has been that evidence should be provided beyond that from biochemical measures, although they have not typically required cardiovascular event trials. Acceptable surrogate indicators of atherosclerosis risk have included measurements of changes in carotid intimal medial thickness and changes in atherosclerotic plaque progression assessed with quantitative coronary angiography or intravascular ultrasound. At least two trials with different methods have been required to insure that the findings are consistent and reproducible.

The recent experience with torcetrapib has stimulated debate about whether such an approach is ideal. As reviewed in Chapter 7 on HDL-C, the development of torcetrapib was stopped because an increased risk of cardiovascular morbidity and mortality was observed in a large outcomes trial. However, no evidence of worsening of carotid intimal medial thickness was observed in a separate trial. This has led some to question whether surrogate measures of atherosclerosis progression should be sufficient evidence to presume efficacy for reducing event risk. In fact, progression of atherosclerosis is only one of several factors that increase the risk of an event. Others include inflammation leading to plaque instability and rupture, the propensity to form an occlusive thrombus on the site of a plaque fissure, and the activity of the fibrinolytic system for dissolving an established clot. Thus, measures of plaque progression are far from perfect indicators of the ultimate impact of a drug on event risk, as risk may be favorably or unfavorably influenced by factors unrelated to plaque development and progression.

The authors remain unconvinced that requiring event trials for all new lipid drugs would best serve public health, although in some instances such a requirement may be reasonable. The approach that the FDA has traditionally taken which is to accept evidence from surrogate indicators in most instances does, in the view of the authors, meet the appropriate regulatory standard of accepting evidence from [6]:

"... adequate and well-controlled clinical trials establishing that the drug product has an effect on a surrogate endpoint that is *reasonably likely*, based on epidemiologic, therapeutic, pathophysiologic, or other evidence, to predict clinical benefit ... " [emphasis added]

Regulatory policy can be influenced unduly by recent or spectacular events and the debates and political pressures that result. As with developing guidelines for treatment, establishing regulatory policy always involves trade-offs and the need to act in the face of imperfect and incomplete information. Finding the right balance between protecting the public from drugs with identifiable adverse effects and maintaining an environment that encourages innovation and does not unnecessarily delay the availability of true medical advances is a difficult and an ever-evolving process.

REFERENCES

[1] Joshi, G.P., Gertler, R. and Fricker, R. (2007) Cardiovascular thromboembolic adverse effects associated with cyclooxygenase-2 selective inhibitors and nonselective antiinflammatory drugs. *Anesthesia and Analgesia*, **105**, 1793–804.

[2] McGettigan, P. and Henry, D. (2006) Cardiovascular risk and inhibition of cyclooxygenase: a systematic review of the observational studies of selective and nonselective inhibitors of cyclooxygenase 2. *The Journal of the American Medical Association*, **296**, 1633–44.

[3] Nissen, S.E., Wolski, K. and Topol, E.J. (2005) Effect of muraglitazar on death and major adverse cardiovascular events in patients with type 2 diabetes mellitus. *The Journal of the American Medical Association*, **294**, 2581–86.

[4] Tanne, J.H. (2006) Pfizer stops clinical trials of heart drug. *British Medical Journal*, **333**, 1237.

[5] U.S. Food and Drug Administration (2007) *Information for Healthcare Professionals*. Nov 19 2007, http://www.fda.gov/CDER/drug/InfoSheets/HCP/rosiglitazone200707HCP.htm.

[6] Orloff, D.G. (2007) Regulatory considerations in the development of high-density lipoprotein therapies. *The American Journal of Cardiology*, **100**(11A), 1QN–14N.

REFERENCES

[1] Hennekens, C.H. and Buring, J.E. (1987) *Epidemiology in Medicine*, (ed S.L. Mayrent), Little, Brown & Company, Boston.

[2] Pocock, S.J. (1983) *Clinical Trials: A Practical Approach*, John Wiley & Sons, Ltd, Chichester.

[3] Appel, L.J., Moore, T.J., Obarzanek, E. *et al*. DASH Collaborative Research Group (1997) A clinical trial of the effects of dietary patterns on blood pressure. *The New England Journal of Medicine*, **336**, 1117–24.

[4] Sauerland, S. and Seiler, C.M. (2005) Role of systematic reviews and meta-analysis in evidence-based medicine. *World Journal of Surgery*, **29**, 582–87.

[5] Feinsten, J.S. (1993) The relationship between socioeconomic status and health: a review of the literature. *The Milbank Quarterly*, **71**, 279–322.

[6] Hemingway, H., Nicholson, A., Stafford, M. *et al*. (1997) The impact of socioeconomic status on health functioning as assessed by the SF-36 questionnaire: the Whitehall II Study. *American Journal of Public Health*, **87**, 1484–90.

[7] Winkleby, M.A., Kraemer, H.C., Ahn, D.K. and Varady, A.N. (1998) Ethnic and socioeconomic differences in cardiovascular disease risk factors: findings for women from the Third National Health and Nutrition Examination Survey, 1988-1994. *The Journal of the American Medical Association*, **280**, 356–62.

[8] Clegg, D.O., Reda, D.J., Harris, C.L. *et al*. (2006) Glucosamine, chondroitin sulfate, and the two in combination for painful knee osteoarthritis. *The New England Journal of Medicine*, **354**, 795–808.

[9] Utian, W.H., Lederman, S.A., Williams, B.M. *et al*. (2004) Relief of hot flushes with new plant-derived 10-component synthetic conjugated estrogens. *Obstetrics and Gynecology*, **103**, 245–53.

[10] Toth, P.P. (2007) The COURAGE Trial: establishing the therapeutic legitimacy of aggressive risk factor management in patients with stable coronary artery disease as an alternative to percutaneous coronary intervention. *Current Atherosclerosis Reports*, **9**, 345–46.

[11] Lipid Research Clinic Program (1984) The lipid research clinics coronary primary prevention trial results. I. Reduction in incidence of coronary heart disease. *The Journal of the American Medical Association,* **251**, 351–64.

[12] Hulley, S., Grady, D., Bush, T. *et al*. Heart and Estrogen/progestin Replacement Study (HERS) Research Group (1998) Randomized trial of estrogen plus progestin for secondary prevention of coronary heart disease in postmenopausal women. *The Journal of the American Medical Association*, **280**, 605–13.

[13] Multiple Risk Factor Intervention Trial Research Group (1982) Multiple risk factor intervention trial. Risk factor changes and mortality results. The Journal of the American Medical Association, 248, 1465–77.

[14] FIELD Investigators (2005) Effects of long-term fenofibrate therapy on cardiovascular events in 9795 people with type 2 diabetes mellitus (the FIELD study): randomised controlled trial. *Lancet*, **366**, 1849–61.

[15] Colhoun, H.M., Betteridge, D.J., Durrington, P.N. *et al*. The CARDS Investigators (2004) Primary prevention of cardiovascular disease with atorvastatin in type 2 diabetes in the Collaborative Atorvastatin Diabetes Study (CARDS): multicentre randomised placebo-controlled trial. *Lancet*, **364**, 685–96.

[16] Marlowe, D.B., Festinger, D.S. and Lee, P.A. (2004) The judge is a key component of drug court. *Drug Court Review*, **4**, 1–34.

[17] Montori, V.M. and Guyatt, G.H. (2001) Intention-to-treat principle. *Canadian Medical Association Journal*, **165**, 1339–41.

11 Case Studies

In this chapter of *Practical Lipid Management*, a series of case studies will be used to illustrate the clinical management of a variety of dyslipidemias in men and women and in patients from different racial and ethnic groups. Emphasis is placed on types of dyslipidemia that are commonly encountered in daily clinical practice. The use of Framingham risk assessment is illustrated. Risk stratified lipoprotein targets are consistent with National Cholesterol Education Program Adult Treatment Panel III (NCEP ATP III) definitions [1]. It must be emphasized that there is always more than one approach that can be used to manage a given clinical presentation. Herein particular attention is given to approaches that are both practical and, whenever possible, evidence-based.

In NCEP ATP III, patients are stratified according to 10-year estimates of risk for a cardiovascular event. If a patient has 0–1 risk factors, they have low risk (10-year risk <5%). If a patient has two or more cardiovascular risk factors (in the absence of coronary heart disease (CHD) or a known risk equivalent), then a Framingham risk score should be calculated so as to determine their lipoprotein target levels. If a patient has CHD or a CHD risk equivalent [diabetes mellitus, abdominal aortic aneurysm (AAA), symptomatic carotid artery disease or a carotid plaque that is >50% obstructive, or peripheral arterial disease (PAD)], then it is not necessary to calculate a Framingham risk score since the individual is classified as high risk. Patients with multiple risk factors with a 10-year Framingham risk score >20% are also defined as having a CHD risk equivalent, thus at high risk for a CHD event. Patients with CHD who smoke, have diabetes mellitus, have had an acute coronary syndrome (ACS), or who have multiple poorly controlled cardiovascular risk factors are considered to be at "very high" risk [2]. These principles are summarized in Figure 11.1.

Framingham risk scoring is a cumulative point scale that depends on age, smoking status, serum total cholesterol (TC) and high-density lipoprotein cholesterol (HDL-C), and systolic blood pressure (BP) (treated or untreated). (See Chapter 3 for more detail.) Although the risk factors are the

Practical Lipid Management: Concepts and Controversies   Peter P. Toth and Kevin C. Maki
© 2008 John Wiley & Sons, Ltd

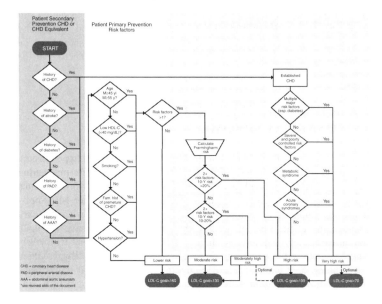

If a patient has established coronary heart disease (CHD), diabetes mellitus, peripheral arterial disease (PAD), abdominal aortic aneurysm (AAA), or a history of stroke, then they are assigned high risk status. If a patient has 0-1 risk factors, then they are low risk and calculation of a Framingham risk score is not necessary. If a patient has 2 or more major CHD risk factors but no evidence of a CHD risk equivalent, then they should undergo risk stratification with a Framingham risk score. Risk stratification defines the LDL-C and non-HDL-C target with therapy. The non-HDL-C goal is simply the LDL-C goal plus 30 mg/dL. If the risk score is >20%, then the patient is high risk and is assigned CHD risk equivalency status. In patients with established CHD, if they have metabolic syndrome, a history of an acute coronary syndrome, multiple poorly controlled risk factors, or still smoke, then they are considered very high risk and have lower, more aggressive optional goals of therapy.

Figure 11.1 Establishing low-density lipoprotein cholesterol (LDL-C) goals. A full-color version of this figure appears in the color plate section of this book. This algorithm, created through the Leadership Council for Cardiovascular Care, is reproduced with permission of Schering Corporation. ©2007 Schering Corporation. All rights reserved.

same, the point scoring system is distinct for men and women. Higher point totals are associated with greater risk over 10 years for a cardiovascular event. Also, no matter how much greater than 60 mg dl^{-1} a patient's serum HDL-C is, it is still only a -1 in Framingham scoring. Consequently, if a patient presents with baseline HDL-C of 80 mg dl^{-1} or even >100 mg dl^{-1}, if he or she has two or more risk factors, the Framingham score should still be calculated in order to determine 10-year projected risk and low-density lipoprotein cholesterol (LDL-C) and non-HDL-C goals. It should not be assumed that very high serum HDL-C levels are cardioprotective in the face of a significant risk factor burden.

CASE ONE: CAD WITH RECENT ACUTE CORONARY SYNDROME

AH is a 63-year-old Caucasian female with a history of CHD, hypertension, hyperlipidemia, and osteoarthritis. She sustained an anterior myocardial infarction (MI) one month ago. She had been smoking 20–30 cigarettes daily for nearly 40 years, but quit immediately following her MI. She is a lifelong homemaker and is neither diabetic nor overweight. Coronary angiography at the time of her MI showed a 99% obstructive lesion in her proximal left anterior descending (LAD) coronary artery with overlying thrombus. Patency of the arterial lumen was reestablished with a drug-eluting stent within 1.5 h of symptom onset. Myocardial salvage was quite good and her current left ventricular ejection fraction (LVEF) is estimated to be 61% based on echocardiographic evaluation. She was noted to have diffuse CHD with lesions ranging from 15–40% in her circumflex, right coronary artery (RCA), and first diagonal branch. None of these lesions warranted stenting. Since placement of her coronary stent she has been free of any signs or symptoms of myocardial ischemia.

The patient's current medications include atorvastatin 10 mg po qd, carvedilol 12.5 mg po bid, aspirin 81 mg po qd, clopidogrel 75 mg po qd, ramipril 10 mg po qd, and acetaminophen 1350 mg po bid. Her BP is 116/70 mmHg and pulse 58 bpm. The lipid profile shows a TC 173 mg dl^{-1}, LDL-C 95 mg dl^{-1}, triglycerides 112 mg dl^{-1}, non-HDL-C 118 mg dl^{-1}, and HDL-C 55 mg dl^{-1}. Her liver function tests (LFTs) reveal no abnormalities. The patient's physical examination is unremarkable.

AH has multivessel CAD with a recent history of an ACS. She meets NCEP criteria for the designation of very high risk. There is no need to calculate her Framingham risk score. LDL-C is the primary target of therapy followed by non-HDL-C. In an effort to reduce her LDL-C to <70 mg dl^{-1} and non-HDL-C <100 mg dl^{-1} (very high risk category), her intake of saturated fat and cholesterol was reduced with the help of a dietitian. She began cardiac rehabilitation to increase her capacity for exercise, she was urged to remain completely abstinent of cigarette smoke (both primary and secondary) and her atorvastatin was increased to 80 mg po qd. This dose of atorvastatin has been shown to be efficacious in reducing risk for cardiovascular events in patients with CAD with or without a history of ACS [3, 4].

Three months after initiating lifestyle modification and intensification of her statin therapy, her TC was 138 mg dl^{-1}, LDL-C was 65 mg dl^{-1}, triglycerides 70 mg dl^{-1}, non-HDL-C 79 mg dl^{-1}, and HDL-C 59 mg dl^{-1}. The patient's serum transaminases remained in normal range and she was not experiencing any symptoms of myopathy. She remained abstinent of cigarette smoke and was walking for between 30 and 45 min daily without precipitating any chest discomfort. She continued to follow-up with her dietitian and maintained a diet low in cholesterol and saturated fat. She was urged to continue her current pharmacologic regimen and to return for routine clinical surveillance in four months.

CASE TWO: PERIPHERAL ARTERIAL DISEASE (PAD)

OR is a 52-year-old African American male who presents to your office complaining of pain in his right buttock, proximal thigh, and calf with ambulation. With rest symptoms gradually resolve. If he begins to ambulate again, symptoms recur after approximately 10 min. He experiences occasional numbness in his feet, but it is not persistent. There has been no tingling or motor weakness. He has seen an internist and a chiropractor both of whom strongly suspected a lumbar radiculopathy. X rays of his lower back and magnetic resonance imaging revealed mild degenerative changes along his spine, but there was no evidence of disk disease, nerve, or spinal cord compression, or of vertebral fracture. Chiropractic manipulation offered no relief in the intensity or the duration of his symptoms. Therapy with a non-steroidal anti-inflammatory medication also did not prevent his episodes of pain.

OR smokes two packs of cigarettes daily. He is an accomplished jazz musician and performs late every evening. The remainder of his review of systems is negative. Physical examination is significant for reduced femoral and pedal pulses on the right side. He has no peripheral edema, dependent rubor, or pedal cyanosis. His musculoskeletal examination as well as gait, coordination, proprioception, and motor strength are normal. His ankle-brachial indices read 0.6 on the right and 1.20 on the left. It is concluded that patient is experiencing claudication secondary to PAD. A magnetic resonance angiogram reveals significant atherosclerotic disease in the right common iliac and the right peroneal arteries. He does not have critical limb ischemia. Screening laboratory studies reveal serum creatinine of 0.9 mg dl^{-1}, normal LFTs and TSH, and a fasting blood sugar (FBS) of 210 mg dl^{-1}. A 2-h glucose tolerance test shows a serum glucose of

270 mg dl^{-1}. His hemoglobin A1c is 8.4%. A lipid profile reveals a TC 206 mg dl^{-1}, LDL-C 130 mg dl^{-1}, triglycerides 170 mg dl^{-1}, non-HDL-C 164 mg dl^{-1}, and HDL-C 42 mg dl^{-1}. Blood pressure is 165/100 mmHg and his 24-h urinary albumin excretion rate is 73 mg.

The patient has symptomatic PAD and does not require calculation of his Framingham risk score. He is by definition categorized as high risk. This patient requires intensive, comprehensive risk factor management since he meets criteria for diabetes mellitus, albuminuria, hypertension, and dyslipidemia. Treadmill stress testing is negative for the precipitation of either chest discomfort or electrocardiographic evidence of myocardial ischemia. The need for cigarette smoking cessation is reviewed in detail. He has tried to quit smoking on multiple occasions but has been unsuccessful. He is started on the nicotinic acetylcholine receptor agonist varenicline in order to reduce both the craving for cigarettes and intensity of nicotine withdrawal. He is taught glucometry, meets with a dietitian, and begins metformin 500 mg po bid. He understands that his target hemoglobin A1c will be <6.5%. He is enrolled in a supervised exercise rehabilitation program and understands the critical need for daily sustained ambulation. In order to treat his hypertension and albuminuria, he is initially treated with losartan 50 mg po qd and hydrochlorothiazide 12.5 mg po qd. His dyslipidemia is treated with simvastatin 40 mg po qd. In addition to treating dyslipidemia, statin therapy in patients with PAD helps to reduce the frequency and intensity of claudication [5]. His target LDL-C and non-HDL-C goals are <100 mg dl^{-1} and <130 mg dl^{-1}, respectively. The patient has no history of peptic ulcer disease and begins aspirin 325 mg po qd.

During the following weeks, his blood sugar responds well to metformin therapy. His metformin dose is increased to 1000 mg po bid and he begins pioglitazone 15 mg po qd. After six weeks, his BP is 147/90 and his losartan is increased to 100 mg dl^{-1}. He is told that his BP target is <130/80 mmHg. Serum creatinine is stable at 0.9 mg dl^{-1}. The patient was able to quit smoking after one month of varenicline therapy. He is advised to continue this for two more months. He is experiencing claudication less frequently and, when it does occur, it resolves more rapidly. He continues to attend sessions with his dietitian and walks daily. His lipid profile has improved significantly, with LDL-C 85 mg dl^{-1}, triglycerides 136 mg dl^{-1}, non-HDL-C 112 mg dl^{-1}, and HDL-C 46 mg dl^{-1}. He is advised to continue his current therapeutic course. Over time, it is hoped that with aggressive risk factor management, he will improve his endothelial dysfunction, reverse his albuminuria, and stabilize/reverse the atherosclerotic disease in his lower extremity and develop collateral arterial flow to further attenuate his claudication.

CASE THREE: PATIENT WITH HETEROZYGOUS FAMILIAL HYPERCHOLESTEROLEMIA

PW is a 39-year-old Caucasian male with a strong family history for CHD and hypercholesterolemia. His mother, maternal grandmother, and three maternal uncles all required revascularization with coronary artery bypass grafting or percutaneous coronary angioplasty by the time they entered into their late 40s and early 50s. His father is 73 and has no history of any form of atherosclerotic disease. PW is an electrical engineer, has no complaints, has no symptoms of coronary ischemia, does not smoke, and he runs three miles daily. He has three younger siblings, none of whom have yet been diagnosed with CHD.

PW has no xanthomas and is physically fit with a normal examination. Waist circumference is 34 in. FBS is 82 mg dl^{-1}, with normal hepatic function panel, TSH, renal indices, and electrocardiogram (ECG). Blood pressure is 105/60 mmHg. Lipid profile shows TC 333 mg dl^{-1}, LDL-C 260 mg dl^{-1}, triglycerides 78 mg dl^{-1}, non-HDL-C 276 mg dl^{-1}, and HDL-C 57 mg dl^{-1}. He is counseled to initiate a therapeutic lifestyle changes (TLC) diet and statin therapy. His Framingham score gives him a 10-year CHD event risk of 3%, which places him in the low risk group. This patient's LDL-C target is <160 mg dl^{-1}. Given the fact that he likely has heterozygous familial hypercholesterolemia and a documented strong family history for premature CHD, it would be prudent to lower his target value further. The patient is started on rosuvastatin 20 mg po qd. After six weeks of therapy, the patient's lipid values include: TC 191 mg dl^{-1}, LDL-C 117 mg dl^{-1}, triglycerides 61 mg dl^{-1}, non-HDL-C 129 mg dl^{-1}, and HDL-C 62 mg dl^{-1}. He is tolerating his dietary modification and drug therapy without adverse side effects and is encouraged to maintain this regimen lifelong so as to reduce his risk for developing CHD.

CASE FOUR: SEVERE HYPERTRIGLYCERIDEMIA

LF is a 45-year-old Hispanic American male who was told by his previous physician that he had severe hypertriglyceridemia. The patient wanted to treat this in a "natural" manner and attempted a low fat diet without success. He has recently moved to the area and notes a history of pancreatitis two years ago. He does not want this to ever occur again as he knows that recurrent pancreatitis can cause chronic pain, diabetes mellitus, and other complications. He wants to try to treat his triglycerides once again.

The patient is not currently experiencing any epigastric or abdominal pain. He is tolerating a general diet. He loves the food from his native Mexico. BP is 135/75 mmHg, pulse 68 bpm, and he is 5′8" with waist circumference of 34 in. He does not smoke but there is a family history of "bad cholesterol" in his four brothers and father. Two of his brothers have also had pancreatitis. There is no family history of premature CHD. His father died of colon cancer at the age of 54. The patient had a colonoscopy one year ago which was unremarkable. Physical examination is normal for age. His serum amylase and lipase are normal. LFTs, renal, and glycemic indices, T4 and TSH, and ECG are all normal. His serum triglycerides are 3500 mg dl^{-1}. HDL-C is 32 mg dl^{-1}. Because his triglycerides are over 400 mg dl^{-1}, his serum LDL-C cannot be calculated using the Friedewald equation. Inspection of his plasma specimen shows that it is milky and turbid.

It is quite likely that this patient has a mutation affecting his activity of the enzyme lipoprotein lipase. This can involve a mutation in the gene for lipoprotein lipase, or it can represent underexpression of the activator of lipoprotein lipase (apoprotein CII) or overexpression of this enzyme's inhibitor, apoprotein CIII. When lipoprotein lipase activity is reduced from either low enzyme mass, or increased inhibition, patients have reduced capacity for triglyceride catabolism. Serum levels of triglycerides can increase to very high levels. Your first priority will be to reduce his serum levels of triglycerides as much as possible in order to prevent additional episodes of pancreatitis. The patient is counseled about a low fat diet and advised to keep a detailed food diary for seven days. He and his wife meet with a dietitian who reviews the diary with them and provides a series of written recommendations on how is diet should be altered. The patient is started on fenofibrate at 145 mg po qd and purified omega-3 fatty acids (Lovaza) at 4.0 g daily. He is advised to follow up in six weeks with a repeat lipid and liver profile.

With medication and dietary changes, his lipid profile shows serum triglyceride of 1400 mg dl^{-1}, HDL-C 36 mg dl^{-1}, and a direct LDL-C of 170 mg dl^{-1}. His triglycerides are still dangerously elevated. The patient is advised to begin pancreatic lipase inhibitor orlistat 120 mg po with each meal. He is cautioned about the possibility of diarrhea and oily stools secondary to impaired fat absorption. After eight weeks of this drug combination, the patient's transaminase levels are normal and serum triglycerides are 275 mg dl^{-1}, TC 262 mg dl^{-1}, HDL-C 38 mg dl^{-1}, and direct LDL-C 165 mg dl^{-1}. His current Framingham risk score is 7%, which places him in the moderate risk group. His serum LDL-C and non-HDL-C targets should be <130 mg dl^{-1} and <160 mg dl^{-1}, respectively. In order to further reduce his serum LDL-C and triglycerides and raise his HDL-C, the patient continues all of his current antilipidemic medications but also begins atorvastatin 10 mg po qd. After eight weeks of therapy he returns to clinic and notes no adverse side effects from his medications. Serum transaminase levels remain normal. His TC is 193 mg dl^{-1}, LDL-C 116 mg dl^{-1}, non-HDL-C 159 mg dl^{-1}, HDL-C 44 mg dl^{-1}, and serum triglycerides 180 mg dl^{-1}. The patient is urged to continue this pharmacologic and lifestyle regimen lifelong.

CASE FIVE: METABOLIC SYNDROME

SG is a 64-year-old Asian Indian female who is referred by her gynecologist for management of multiple cardiovascular risk factors. At the time of her annual gynecologic evaluation, the patient was noted to be obese and have a BP of 146/92, pulse 88, FBS 115 mg dl^{-1}, normal TSH and renal indices, and normal LFTs. A 2-h glucose tolerance test reveals a glucose value of 185 mg dl^{-1}. A fasting lipid profile shows TC 217 mg dl^{-1}, LDL-C 122 mg dl^{-1}, triglycerides 305 mg dl^{-1}, non-HDL-C 183 mg dl^{-1}, and HDL-C 34 mg dl^{-1}. The patient smokes 20 cigarettes daily. The patient's waist circumference is 39 in. Baseline ECG is normal with no evidence for myocardial ischemia, arrhythmia, or bundle branch block. The patient's Framingham risk score is 11%, which places SG in the moderately high risk group. Her lipid targets include LDL-C and non-HDL-C of <130 mg dl^{-1} and <160 mg dl^{-1}, respectively (or, based on the NCEP update of 2004, she has optional, more stringent goals of <100 mg dl^{-1} and <130 mg dl^{-1}, respectively).

SG meets diagnostic criteria for all five components of the metabolic syndrome. She has a waist circumference >35 in., BP >130/85 mmHg, FBS >100 mg dl^{-1}, HDL-C <50 mg dl^{-1}, and triglycerides >150 mg dl^{-1}. This places her at increased risk for both diabetes mellitus and cardiovascular disease. While it might be assumed that she is high risk, her Framingham risk score places her at moderately high risk for CHD. Because of her age and the fact that she smokes, it would be in the patient's best interest to treat her atherogenic lipoproteins to the more stringent target levels suggested by the NCEP [2]. It is imperative that SG quit smoking. In addition to inducing endothelial dysfunction, and accelerating atherogenesis, smoking also promotes insulin resistance by increasing systemic expression of tumor necrosis factor-alpha. The patient is determined to quit by herself and decides to go "cold turkey." She is advised to try to lose 20 lbs in an effort to reduce her insulin resistance and to begin an exercise regimen. She thinks she would enjoy walking in the pool at the local YMCA and is willing to do this for 20–30 min daily. She is a vegetarian and receives nutritional counseling because of the high starch/carbohydrate content of her diet. Because of her risk factor profile, age, and chronic smoking status, she undergoes a stress echocardiogram in order to ensure that it is safe for her to begin daily exercise. This revealed no electrocardiographic abnormalities or any impairment in ventricular wall motion. Her LVEF is estimated at 70%. An albumin/creatinine spot ratio is normal and her 24-h albumin secretory rate is 17 mg. She is started on aspirin 81 mg po qd, enalapril 20 mg po qd, and pravastatin 40 mg po qd.

After three weeks of therapy, her BP decreases to 134/85 mmHg. She has quit smoking. She is exercising in the pool six days per week and has lost 3 lbs. Hydrochlorothiazide 12.5 mg po qd is added to her antihypertensive regimen. She is advised to follow-up in three weeks. At time of follow-up, her BP is 125/80 mmHg. Despite having quit smoking, she has lost another 4 lbs. She notes that she feels better than she has in years. Her lipid profile is improved with TC 171 mg dl^{-1}, LDL-C 82 mg dl^{-1}, triglycerides 230 mg dl^{-1}, non-HDL-C 128, and HDL-C 43 mg dl^{-1}. The patient has had a disproportionate rise in HDL-C most likely secondary to the combination of statin therapy as well as smoking cessation and other forms of lifestyle modification (weight loss, dietary modification). The patient's HDL-C, and triglycerides remain abnormal. In an effort to further raise her HDL-C and decrease her triglycerides, fenofibrate 145 mg po qd is added to her pharmacologic regimen. After six weeks of combination lipid-lowering therapy and continued lifestyle modification, the patient's lipid profile is now normal: TC 158 mg dl^{-1}, LDL-C 78 mg dl^{-1}, triglycerides 147 mg dl^{-1}, non-HDL-C 107 mg dl^{-1}, and HDL-C 51 mg dl^{-1}.

CASE SIX: INTOLERANCE OF INTERMEDIATE-DOSE STATIN THERAPY

IF is a 59-year-old Caucasian male with stable CHD. IF does not have diabetes mellitus, metabolic syndrome, history of an ACS, or any symptoms of myocardial ischemia. He has been treated with multiple statins but the only one he has not experienced myalgias with is rosuvastatin 5 mg po qd. Drug interactions, thyroid dysfunction, muscle trauma, baseline myopathy, and electrolyte disturbances have all been ruled out. His LDL-C is 115 mg dl^{-1}, triglycerides 95 mg dl^{-1}, and HDL-C 52 mg dl^{-1}. In an effort to further reduce his LDL-C to <100 mg dl^{-1}, rosuvastatin is increased to 10 mg po qd. Within 10 days he returns to clinic complaining of diffuse myalgias. His serum creatine phosphokinase (CPK) level is 95 IU l^{-1}, which is normal. He has no objective evidence for motor weakness. After decreasing his rosuvastatin to 5 mg po qd, his myalgias resolve within five days. The patient is then started on ezetimibe therapy in combination with rosuvastatin. After six weeks, his LDL-C decreases to 91 mg dl^{-1}, triglycerides are 90 mg dl^{-1}, and HDL-C is 54 mg dl^{-1}. He is not experiencing any myalgias and LFTs remain normal.

Ezetimibe provides patients with an acceptable alternative to statin titration when additional LDL-C reduction is needed in order for a patient to achieve their NCEP goals. The addition of ezetimibe to any given statin dose is equivalent to three statin titration steps. Assuming that each doubling of a statin's dose reduces LDL-C by approximately 6% (the "rule of sixes"), this patient would have required two titration steps (5 → 10 → 20 mg) in order to reduce LDL-C to <100 mg dl^{-1}. The addition of ezetimibe helped the patient achieve his LDL-C goal without exacerbating myalgia.

CASE SEVEN: PATIENT WITH ISCHEMIC STROKE

JK is a 71-year-old African American female with a history of an ischemic cerebrovascular accident (CVA) two years ago. At that time she had evidence of a single atheromatous plaque in her right internal carotid artery that was 30% obstructive and without ulceration. The left carotid arterial system showed some intimal thickening but no obvious atheromatous plaquing. At the time of her CVA she developed left upper extremity weakness with tingling. She could not grasp and had reduced motor strength in her wrist and forearm. None of her cranial nerves were affected. She had no cognitive impairment. She experienced complete recovery of motor function over the course of three days. Magnetic resonance imaging of her brain revealed no evidence of infarction with the parietal cortex. She was fully ambulatory and had full capacity to perform her activities of daily living. She was started on a daily aspirin (325 mg).

The patient's hypertension was well controlled with ramipril 10 mg po qd and amlodipine 10 mg po qd. At the time of her CVA her lipid profile revealed LDL-C 98 mg dl^{-1}, triglycerides 110 mg dl^{-1}, and HDL-C 52 mg dl^{-1}. She had smoked for 30 years but quit at the time of her CVA. She does not have diabetes and she is lean with a waist circumference of 27 in. She is active and is a committed local church leader. She wants everything possible to be done to reduce her risk of having another CVA. The first one frightened her considerably. A repeat lipid profile shows an LDL-C of 96 mg dl^{-1}, triglycerides 136 mg dl^{-1}, and HDL-C 50 mg dl^{-1}. Chest X ray, ECG, and physical examination are normal. Carotid upstrokes are brisk and she has no carotid, abdominal, or femoral bruits. Her glycemic, renal, and thyroid indices are normal. Her BP is 118/73 mmHg and she is taking her antihypertensive medications. A repeat carotid duplex ultrasound study confirms the presence of a 30% lesion in her right internal carotid artery. There is also a new 20% lesion in her left carotid bulb with no apparent fissuring or ulceration.

Given the fact that she has established atherosclerotic disease in her carotid system, it is quite reasonable to consider statin therapy even though her lipid profile meets NCEP targets for a high risk patient. Many of the statin trials have shown reductions in the risk for ischemic stroke [6]. In the Stroke Prevention by Aggressive Reduction in Cholesterol Levels (SPARCL) trial, atorvastatin dosed at 80 mg daily significantly reduced risk of recurrent ischemic stroke [7]. Since the patient requests that maximal therapy be undertaken to reduce risk of a second stroke, she is started on atorvastatin 10 mg daily and then titrated to 80 mg daily over the course of four months. She is tolerating the medication without adverse side effects. On 80 mg of atorvastatin daily her LDL-C is 50 mg dl^{-1}, triglycerides 87 mg dl^{-1}, and HDL-C 57 mg dl^{-1}. It is hoped that with these lipid levels and continued good control of her BP, her carotid artery plaque will not only stabilize, but also perhaps regress. She is advised to return for follow up blood chemistries every six months.

CASE EIGHT: PATIENT WITH CHEST PAIN ON GEMFIBROZIL

YC is a 67-year old Asian male on gemfibrozil therapy for the past 10 years because of hypertriglyceridemia and low HDL-C. At the time of initiating fibrate therapy and dietary modification, his lipid profile shows LDL-C 105 mg dl^{-1}, triglycerides 320 mg dl^{-1}, and HDL-C 34 mg dl^{-1}. After three months of therapy LDL-C was 118 mg dl^{-1}, triglycerides 162 mg dl^{-1}, and HDL-C 39 mg dl^{-1}. The patient is lean and does not meet criteria for metabolic syndrome as his BP is 124/68 mmHg, FBS is 88 mg dl^{-1}, and his waist circumference is 28 in. He presents to clinic because of episodic chest pain for the past two weeks. He thought at first it was indigestion because it could be accompanied by nausea at times. However, in the past three days, he is experiencing substernal pressure, interscapular discomfort, diaphoresis, and occasional radiation of pain into his neck and left jaw. An ECG reveals ST-segment depressions inferiorly and anteriorly. YC is admitted to the hospital where his initial myocardial markers (troponin, myoglobin) are negative for evidence of acute myocardial injury. He undergoes cardiac catheterization and is noted to have a tight 90% stenosis along his mid LAD and another flow-limiting lesion with 95% stenosis along his proximal RCA. Both of these lesions are successfully stented with drug-eluting stents. He experiences no recurrence of chest or interscapular discomfort and he feels well.

A lipid profile in hospital shows a TC 163 mg dl^{-1}, LDL-C 116 mg dl^{-1}, triglycerides 148, non-HDL-C 125 mg dl^{-1}, and HDL 37 mg dl^{-1}. The patient has been revascularized and given his recent history of unstable angina, meets criteria for ACS and very high risk status. His LDL-C and non-HDL-C should be reduced to <70 mg dl^{-1} and <100 mg dl^{-1}. Because statin therapy is clearly indicated in this case, gemfibrozil should be discontinued. When gemfibrozil is coadministered with a statin, the gemfibrozil can reduce the glucuronidation and elimination of the statin, leading to increased risk for rhabdomyolysis and hepatotoxicity [8, 9]. The gemfibrozil is discontinued and fenofibrate 145 mg po qd is started in order to control serum triglycerides and raise HDL-C. The patient is also simultaneously started on simvastatin 20 mg po qd. In addition to lipid-lowering medication, he is also started on Lopressor 25 mg po bid, aspirin 81 mg po qd, clopidogrel 75 mg po qd, Lovaza 1000 mg po qd, and nitroglycerin (NTG) 0.4 mg sublingual PRN. After six weeks of therapy, YC's ECG is normal. He has not had to use any NTG. BP is 105/60 and pulse 60 bpm. LFTs remain normal. His lipid profile shows: TC 128 mg dl^{-1}, LDL-C 60 mg dl^{-1}, triglycerides

116 mg dl^{-1}, non-HDL-C 84 mg dl^{-1}, and HDL-C 44 mg dl^{-1}. He is advised to return to clinic for follow up in three months.

CASE NINE: LOW HDL-C IN A PATIENT WITH STABLE CHD AND EARLY CAROTID DISEASE

AF is a 72-year-old Caucasian female with stable CHD and early evidence of carotid artery disease as evidenced by increased carotid intima media thickness bilaterally on a carotid duplex ultrasonography scan. The patient underwent a three-vessel coronary artery bypass grafting procedure three years ago. She has had lifelong low HDL-C and never smoked. She does not have diabetes mellitus and does not meet criteria for metabolic syndrome. AF is currently on fluvastatin 40 mg po qd with LDL-C 77 mg dl^{-1}, triglycerides 76 mg dl^{-1}, and HDL 29 mg dl^{-1}. She walks daily for 45 min with her husband. She is active and is free of any symptoms suggestive of myocardial ischemia. She has tried to raise her HDL-C through lifestyle modification but has been unsuccessful.

The addition of fibrate therapy would be inappropriate in this patient given the fact that she does not have hypertriglyceridemia. Her LDL-C is at target value and titration of her fluvastatin to 80 mg po qd would be unlikely to raise her HDL-C significantly. She is advised to begin Niaspan (extended-release niacin) at 500 mg po at bedtime. The patient understands that of all the currently available medications, niacin supplementation has the greatest capacity to increase serum levels of HDL-C. One potential difficulty of niacin therapy is its ability to activate prostaglandin D$_2$ biosynthesis in the skin, leading to dermal vasodilatation and flushing. She is told that this does not constitute an allergic reaction. After a period of habituation, the flushing does resolve. She is advised to take her 325 mg tablet of aspirin 1-h before taking her Niaspan in an effort to prevent flushing. She is also carefully advised to not substitute over the counter niacin for Niaspan because of its variable purity and potential contamination with nicotinamide adenine dinucleotide, which is toxic to the liver at high doses.

The patient calls five days later noting that during three of the previous five nights she has had flushing that caused a feeling of intense heat, some pruritus, and dyspepsia. She is advised to take aspirin 1 h before supper and to take Niaspan with supper. This improves her symptoms considerably and within seven days she is no longer experiencing flushing. She denies any myalgias. After one month her Niaspan is increased to 1000 mg daily. After three months of Niaspan at this dose combined with her fluvastatin therapy, her LDL-C is 65 mg dl^{-1}, triglycerides 45 mg dl^{-1}, and HDL is 41 mg dl^{-1}. LFTs remain normal. Her Niaspan is titrated further over the next three months to 2.0 g daily. She understands that at this dose of niacin, not only will her lipid profile improve further, but her risk of acute coronary events [10], need for bypass surgery [11], and risk for progression of carotid artery disease [12] will also be beneficially impacted. Moreover, it is likely that her serum HDL-C will continue to increase for an additional 9–12 months [12]. After 12 months of combination therapy, her HDL-C has increased to 53 mg dl^{-1}. She has habituated to the Niaspan and has no manifestations of toxicity.

CASE TEN: STATIN DRUG INTERACTION WITH HEPATOTOXICITY

EM is a 47-year-old African American female with hypertension and hyper-lipidemia. She had poorly controlled hypertension for a number of years. On presentation her BP is 185/110 and pulse 92 bpm. She notes that both of her parents and all of her siblings have severe hypertension. An echocardiogram reveals left atrial enlargement and significant left ventricular hypertrophy (LVH) with an estimated LVEF of 76%. Her EKG confirms LVH with spik-ing QRS complexes anteriorly, but she does not have an arrhythmia nor is there any evidence of ischemia. EM has been postmenopausal for three years, smokes approximately 10 cigarettes daily, FBS is 96 mg dl^{-1}, waist circumference is 33 in., renal indices are normal, and her physical exami-nation is unremarkable except for the presence of an S3 gallop on cardiac examination. Her rate of urinary albumin secretion is 21 mg day^{-1}. Her lipid profile shows TC 274 mg dl^{-1}, LDL-C 195 mg dl^{-1}, triglycerides 120 mg dl^{-1}, non-HDL-C 219 mg dl^{-1}, and HDL-C 55 mg dl^{-1}. Her 10-year Framingham risk score is 14%, which places EM in the range of moderately high risk. Given the severity of her hypertension and her smok-ing history, her lipid goals are set to the more stringent target of LDL-C <100 mg dl^{-1}. She is started on lisinopril 20 mg po qd, hydrochlorothiazide 12.5 mg po qd, extended-release metoprolol 100 mg po qd, aspirin 81 mg po qd, and simvastatin 40 mg po qd.

After one month of therapy the patient's BP is 150/91 mmHg and pulse 78 bpm. Her serum creatinine is stable at 0.8 mg dl^{-1}. Her lisinopril is increased to 40 mg po qd and her other medications are continued. After six weeks of simvastatin therapy, her LDL-C was 112 mg dl^{-1}, triglycerides 98 mg dl^{-1}, and HDL-C 58 mg dl^{-1}. LFTs remained normal. Her simvas-tatin was increased to 80 mg po qd and she was advised to return to clinic for follow up in six weeks. At that time, her BP was 138/85 mmHg with stable serum creatinine. TC was 175 mg dl^{-1}, LDL-C 98 mg dl^{-1}, triglyc-erides 90 mg dl^{-1}, non-HDL-C 116 mg dl^{-1}, and HDL-C 59 mg dl^{-1}. She was advised to remain on all of her medications and follow-up in six months with repeat lipid and liver profiles.

After six months of therapy, the patient's lipid profile was stable and at target levels. However, her serum alanine aminotransferase (ALT) and aspartate aminotransferase (AST) levels increased to 1276 and 1050 U l^{-1}, respectively. She felt well and was not experiencing any myalgias, right upper quadrant pain, impaired appetite, nausea, or malaise. She was asked if she had been started on any new medications by another physician. She replied that three months ago she was admitted to the hospital by a cardiologist for atrial fibrillation. She notes that she underwent successful cardioversion and was started on a new medication for heart rhythm disturbances. She was placed on amiodarone 200 mg po bid. It is well documented that in patients treated with amiodarone or verapamil, the dose of simvastatin should not exceed 20 mg dl^{-1} (see also package insert for simvastatin) [13]. At the time of initiating amiodarone, her cardiologist should have switched her to another statin, such as rosuvastatin or atorvastatin, which are not known to interact with amiodarone. The patient's simvastatin was discontinued and her LFTs were monitored every two weeks. Her transaminitis steadily improved with decreasing ALT and AST values. Within two months her LFTs were back within normal range. She was treated with rosuvastatin 20 mg po qd with no subsequent toxicity and her lipoprotein targets were achieved.

CASE ELEVEN: PATIENT WITH DYSLIPIDEMIA AND HISTORY OF RHABDOMYOLYSIS

CD is a 58-year-old Caucasian male with a history of statin-induced rhabdomyolysis. He has no history of any type of atherosclerotic disease. After eight weeks of statin therapy, he developed severe, diffuse, escalating myalgias. He was immediately evaluated and found to have diffuse muscle tenderness with motor weakness in his lower extremities. He had myoglobinuria and serum CPK level was 24 500 U l^{-1}. He was immediately hospitalized and provided with all manner of supportive care including intravenous hydration, analgesia, statin cessation, and electrolyte management. Over the course of the following two days his serum CPK level peaked at 45 000 U l^{-1} and he developed renal failure. He was dialyzed for one week until his renal function recovered. With aggressive physical therapy he regained full motor capacity with no residual deficit or myalgia. The patient understood that this was a potential complication of statin therapy and was grateful it was recognized and treated in an expeditious manner. Subsequent neurologic evaluation revealed no evidence for underlying congenital myopathy or mitochondrial disorder.

The patient's father died of an MI at the age of 56. He is anxious about his cholesterol profile, which shows TC 234 mg dl^{-1}, LDL-C 168 mg dl^{-1}, triglyceride 136 mg dl^{-1}, and HDL-C 39 mg dl^{-1}. He refuses to try another statin and it is agreed that he is a high risk for recurrent rhabdomyolysis. His hypertension is controlled on candesartan, hydrochlorothiazide, and diltiazem. Without medication his BP is 170/95 mmHg, with medication it is 127/78 mmHg. He does not have diabetes and does not smoke. He swims for 45 min four days weekly. He does not have thyroid dysfunction or residual renal compromise. CD's 10-year-old Framingham risk score is 15%, which places him in the moderately high risk group.

If possible, CD agrees that it would be optimal to reduce his LDL <100 mg dl^{-1} and raise his HDL-C above 40 mg dl^{-1}. The patient is treated with ezetimibe 10 mg po qd. In six weeks his LDL-C decreases to 128 mg dl^{-1} and his HDL-C is 41 mg dl^{-1}. Triglycerides are modestly reduced to 121 mg dl^{-1}. He is tolerating the ezetimibe well and without any myalgia or LFT abnormalities. In order to reduce his LDL-C further, the patient is given adjuvant therapy with the bile acid binding resin colesevelam hydrochloride 1250 mg po tid with meals. He understands that because colesevelam has no systemic absorption, it is not associated with any risk for myopathy [14]. After eight weeks of combination therapy, his LDL-C is 96 mg dl^{-1}, triglycerides 128 mg dl^{-1}, and HDL-C 42 mg dl^{-1}. He is tolerating his lipid-lowering regimen with no myalgia, proximal weakness, or sensory neuropathy. LFTs remain normal.

CASE TWELVE: STATIN-INDUCED MYALGIA WITHOUT MYOPATHY

OC is a 65-year-old Hispanic female with diabetes mellitus, hypertension, and dyslipidemia. She has no clinical manifestations of atherosclerotic disease and is highly functional. Her most recent hemoglobin A_{1C} is 6.3% and BP on multiple antihypertensive agents is 115/62 mmHg. She has no renal or thyroid dysfunction. Her cardiologist is requesting a second opinion because he has attempted to treat her dyslipidemia with four different statins, but has had to discontinue all of them due to rapid onset diffuse myalgias occasionally accompanied by subjective proximal motor weakness. Serum CPK levels are routinely less than 75 U l^{-1} and neurologic evaluation is also routinely normal. Without treatment the patient's TC is 231 mg dl^{-1}, LDL-C 142 mg dl^{-1}, triglycerides 205 mg dl^{-1}, and HDL-C is 48 mg dl^{-1}.

OC's lipid profile is clearly abnormal for a patient with diabetes mellitus, a CHD risk equivalent. Statin-induced myalgia and myopathy are complex phenomena and arise from a heterogeneous set of etiologies, including autoimmune, mitochondrial, and isoprenoid-dependent biochemical changes within myocytes [15]. Myalgias are clearly a complication of statin therapy and can occur in up to 15% of patients enrolled in community-based cohorts. There is some evidence that at least in some patients, a deficiency of coenzyme Q10 may underlie statin-induced myalgia [16]. It was recently suggested by Marcoff and Thompson that initiating a trial of coenzyme Q10 in patients with statin-induced myalgia was reasonable given that there are no known toxic effects of coenzyme Q10 supplementation and it might help to resolve myalgia and facilitate compliance with statin therapy. Given OC's high risk status, she elected to proceed with this approach. She was advised to take coenzyme Q10 200 mg daily for three weeks and then begin rosuvastatin 2.5 mg daily. She was also told to immediately report any muscle symptoms that might suggest recurrence of myalgia. OC tolerated this combination quite well. After six weeks of therapy, her LDL-C decreased to 106 mg dl^{-1}. Her rosuvastatin was increased to 5 mg po qd and she was to continue her coenzyme Q10 supplementation for as long as she remained on statin therapy. After six weeks of therapy with the 5 mg dose, her LDL-C decreased to 78 mg dl^{-1}, triglycerides were 153 mg dl^{-1}, and her HDL was 54 mg dl^{-1}. She continued to be free of any myopathy symptoms.

REFERENCES

[1] Expert Panel on Detection, Evaluation, and Treatment of High Blood Cholesterol in Adults (2001) Executive summary of the third report of The National Cholesterol Education Program (NCEP) Expert Panel on Detection, Evaluation, and Treatment of High Blood Cholesterol in Adults (Adult Treatment Panel III). *The Journal of the American Medical Association*, **285**, 2486–97.

[2] Grundy, S.M., Cleeman, J.I., Merz, C.N. *et al.* (2004) Implications of recent clinical trials for the National Cholesterol Education Program Adult Treatment Panel III Guidelines. *Circulation*, **110**, 227–39.

[3] Cannon, C.P., Braunwald, E., McCabe, C.H. *et al.* (2004) Intensive versus moderate lipid lowering with statins after acute coronary syndromes. *The New England Journal of Medicine*, **350**, 1495–504.

[4] LaRosa, J.C., Grundy, S.M., Waters, D.D. *et al.* (2005) Intensive lipid lowering with atorvastatin in patients with stable coronary disease. *The New England Journal of Medicine*, **352**, 1425–35.

[5] The Scandinavian Simvastatin Survival Study Group (1994) Randomised trial of cholesterol lowering in 4444 patients with coronary heart disease: the Scandinavian Simvastatin Survival Study (4S). *Lancet*, **344**, 1383–89.

[6] Armani, A. and Toth, P.P. (2007) SPARCL: the glimmer of statins for stroke risk reduction. *Current Atherosclerosis Reports*, **9**, 347–51.

[7] Amarenco, P., Bogousslavsky, J., Callahan, A. *et al.* (2006) High-dose atorvastatin after stroke or transient ischemic attack. *The New England Journal of Medicine*, **355**, 549–59.

[8] Prueksaritanont, T., Tang, C., Qiu, Y. *et al.* (2002) Effects of fibrates on metabolism of statins in human hepatocytes. *Drug Metabolism and Disposition*, **30**, 1280–87.

[9] Prueksaritanont, T., Zhao, J.J., Ma, B. *et al.* (2002) Mechanistic studies on metabolic interactions between gemfibrozil and statins. *The Journal of Pharmacology and Experimental Therapeutics*, **301**, 1042–51.

[10] Brown, B.G., Zhao, X.Q., Chait, A. *et al.* (2001) Simvastatin and niacin, antioxidant vitamins, or the combination for the prevention of coronary disease. *The New England Journal of Medicine*, **345**, 1583–92.

[11] The Coronary Drug Project Research Group (1975) Clofibrate and niacin in coronary heart disease. *The Journal of the American Medical Association*, **231**, 360–81.

[12] Taylor, A.J., Sullenberger, L.E., Lee, H.J. *et al.* (2004) Arterial biology for the investigation of the treatment effects of reducing cholesterol (ARBITER) 2: a double-blind, placebo-controlled study of extended-release niacin on atherosclerosis progression in secondary prevention patients treated with statins. *Circulation*, **110**, 3512–17.

[13] de Lemos, J.A., Blazing, M.A., Wiviott, S.D. *et al.* (2004) Early intensive vs a delayed conservative simvastatin strategy in patients with acute coronary syndromes: phase Z of the A to Z trial. *The Journal of the American Medical Association*, **292**, 1307–16.

[14] Armani, A. and Toth, P.P. (2006) Colesevelam hydrochloride in the management of dyslipidemia. *Expert Review of Cardiovascular Therapy*, **4**, 283–91.

[15] Harper, C.R. and Jacobson, T.A. (2007) The broad spectrum of statin myopathy: from myalgia to rhabdomyolysis. *Current Opinion in Lipidology*, **18**, 401–8.

[16] Marcoff, L. and Thompson, P.D. (2007) The role of coenzyme Q10 in statin-associated myopathy: a systematic review. *Journal of the American College of Cardiology*, **49**, 2231–37.

Index

Note: Page references in *italics* refer to Figures; those in **bold** refer to Tables

Practical Lipid Management: Concepts and Controversies   Peter P. Toth and Kevin C. Maki
© 2008 John Wiley & Sons, Ltd